DETOX
Your Life

Also by Jane Scrivner
Detox Yourself
Detox Your Mind
The Little Book of Detox

DETOX
Your Life

JANE SCRIVNER

PIATKUS

To Kevin, thank you.

My thanks to everyone at Piatkus: Judy, Rachel, Jane, Jana,
Heather, and everyone I haven't yet met but speak to
often. Thank you for continuing to support my ideas and
generally leaving me alone to get on with it.
And thank you to all my friends who have never failed to
encourage me in these endeavours.

© 1999 Jane Scrivner

First published in 1999 by
Judy Piatkus (Publishers) Ltd
5 Windmill Street
London W1P 1HF

For the latest news and information
on all our titles, visit our new website at
www.piatkus.co.uk

The moral rights of the author have been asserted
A catalogue record for this book is available from the British Library

ISBN 0-7499-2028-9

Designed by Paul Saunders

Typeset by Action Publishing Technology Limited, Gloucester
Printed and bound in Great Britain by Mackays of Chatham PLC

Contents

Introduction

The *Detox Your Life* programme is an amalgamation of techniques which are designed to leave you stunningly detoxed and refreshingly raring to go.

Detox Yourself is about ridding your body of all the waste and toxins which have accumulated over the years. Foodstuffs that are not entirely good for you or that your body is unable to completely assimilate, pollution and chemicals are eliminated and cleansed from your system.

Following a detox plan means that, as well as getting rid of the waste, you are feeding your body with nutrients that it can use and convert into fuel and energy. It is about eliminating all the foods that have a negative effect and including all the foods that positively improve your health and energy.

Detox Your Mind is about ridding your mind of all the stresses and strains of everyday living, sorting out all the lingering worries and problems that you hold in your head and doing something about them. Detoxing your mind changes negatives to positives and makes you see things differently. Problems disappear and return newly dressed as opportunities or challenges.

Detox Your Life applies all the mental and physical detox techniques to your life and then helps you use the findings to see where you want to go. It is about choosing your personal priorities and carrying them out in the way you want.

Detoxing your life is *not* about being selfish or getting your own way to the detriment of others. *Detox Your Life* is about making yourself the most important thing in your life, about creating your own best environment so that being there for others is easy. It is about getting what you truly want.

Our personal and professional lives can be incredibly stimulating, rewarding and satisfying. If they go right, people say that we are 'lucky' or that we have been 'blessed with good fortune'. Yet these comments are merely ways of ignoring the fact that we planned, worked hard and made the best of all the opportunities that came our way, while playing down or overcoming all the problems. Detoxing your life is about deciding what is important and what is not, and then putting the plans into place that will make the good bits happen and the bad bits disappear, or at least make them easier to deal with. It is about having a vision of where you are going and then getting there.

Detoxing your life needs a lot of honesty, a willingness to change and some positive hard work – and then you can achieve anything you truly want. Detoxing your life gives you more freedom to move forward – go for it!

1

How to Use This Book

THE COOKIE JAR THEORY

'If the cookie jar is empty then you can't give them cookies.'

Imagine yourself as a cookie jar. Your jar is full of freshly baked chocolate chip, ginger, orange spice, cinnamon, white chocolate, blueberry, raisin, walnut, coffee and oatmeal cookies. They are warm, highly nutritious – despite their yumminess! – and simply delicious. You love these cookies because you baked them yourself; you feel fulfilled because you have created something and now you can share them with anyone who wants them.

Letting people tuck into these cookies is immensely pleasing. Their hands lift the lid; the smell is wonderful and stimulates the taste buds, the texture is crunchy and crumbly, and the flavour travels from the mouth-watering first bite right through the body until the last crumb. They are pleasing and satisfying; they fill you up and they provide energy to keep you going for the rest of the day.

As the cookies are eaten and enjoyed, you are able to replace them by simply baking a new batch each evening and then placing these in your own personal jar. This is not tiring because it gives you pleasure to bake and see how much everyone enjoys them. You and your life are in cookie heaven.

Now, several weeks later, your cookies have gained a reputation. They are still everything they were before and you still put as much love and attention into them but they are going faster and faster, and you have a job to keep replacing them. Your oven isn't big enough to bake the batch sizes you need to and the hands are dipping into the jar without even taking time to taste the cookie. Some people are even taking a handful of cookies and passing them on to friends! It is OK though because the cookies are still of a high standard – everyone is getting a top-notch cookie. No one would ever know that you are exhausted because it is taking you much more time to replenish the rapidly disappearing stocks. And no one realises that you need some time off because whenever they lift the lid and reach for a cookie, you have made sure that there are plenty to go around – despite the damage to your own health and quality of life.

Six months after they first tasted your cookies, the troops are getting restless. The jar is not always full and when it is it only has one or two flavours, and some of them are a little overcooked or, worse still, a touch too soggy. You have resorted to getting up early to fit in more baking, and you are going to bed tired because you have to spend more of your time thinking up new flavours or looking at new shapes to keep them happy. To keep your sanity, you decide to make one flavour and hope that this will satisfy all. You also decide to make just a few and if they run out or go stale then so be it. Now you realise that you no longer bake with loving care and attention; you simply bake to satisfy the demand for the cookies. They are not even your cookies any more – they have become public property.

The cookie eaters can taste all these changes and they don't like them. They complain: 'Why can't we have cookies like we used to? Why can't we have all the flavours? Why aren't there enough? Why don't you like baking them any more? What has gone wrong? Why is the cookie jar empty?'

If you relate the cookie jar theory to your own life it probably sounds all too familiar. If you do not feel fully replenished and satisfied yourself, you do not have the resources to give out help, time and understanding to other people. If you are not happy with your life, giving away the bits of it that are going well and supplying you with energy to other people will leave you depleted and drained. If no one is putting back into your cookie jar, how can you offer cookies to anyone else? The best person to put back into your jar is *you*. You can replenish, revive, invigorate, satisfy and grow yourself because you are the only person who truly knows what you do and don't want to happen in your life.

Detoxing your life is the natural next step. This book will help you measure, weigh up, evaluate and decide on all aspects of your life. It will empower you to get rid of the stuff you don't want, stop doing the things you don't want to do, and stop living just to satisfy others. It will help you get rid of the negative and concentrate, build and capitalise on the positive.

GETTING STARTED

Warning: This detox programme could seriously improve your life . . .

For the most part we are born, grow up, and live our lives to the best of our ability. Without a great deal of forward planning or even thought as to what we want for ourselves, we get older, look back on our lives, see all the things we have done, regret all the things we haven't done, and then we die. This is completely normal behaviour. It has gone on for years and years and will continue for years to come.

Now, take an important event or occurrence in life and apply the same approach. Let's take starting a new business. Imagine saying to your parents or friends or bank manager that you have an idea for a new business and you are just going to have a go and spend all your money on it, open the doors for trading and hope you get some customers. Or let's take getting married. You meet someone, they seem OK but you have only known them for a week or so, you book the church for the next available date and then invite a whole load of friends and tie the knot. In either case ARE YOU CRAZY?! No planning, no analysis, no getting to know each other, no profit and loss, no budget forecast, no business plan, no guest list, no family consultation, no checking if this is what you both want, no meeting his parents, no job satisfaction, no aims and goals, no looking to the future, no thought, *no idea of what you really want and what is best for you?*

We wouldn't dream of starting a new business without writing a business plan and we wouldn't dream of getting married without making plans for the future. Yet we happily run our daily lives with no idea if we are getting the best we can for ourselves. We accept 'second best' as the norm.

Even if you do nothing but write out your mission statement and your six key tasks (see Chapter 2), you will still have your own personal guide to your life that you can consult. You will have a clear view of all the things you have discovered, all the things you have to work with, and all the things you will gradually let go of until they are no longer part of your life.

In your mind you will have written the manual for [insert your own name] and how you work.

Completing the 25 action steps should physically take about half an hour of your day for each of the detox days. That means that you will be actually writing or making notes on your computer for just 30 minutes a day. (You will probably think about this for a great deal longer than 30 minutes or even 30 days but this is just the beginning of the Detox Your Life process.)

Detoxing your life isn't about making your life perfect and squeaky clean, but it is about knowing what you want for yourself and creating the best opportunities for it to happen. Making your life better for you overall is what detoxing your life is about. Just becoming aware of your own life and how it works is going to be fairly amazing.

So, each day, set aside some time: on the bus into work; in the kitchen during the baby's afternoon nap; with a cup of cocoa in bed before switching the light off; in the sandwich bar at lunch; at the weekend after reading the Sunday papers; in the launderette whilst your smalls are drying.

You will need a pen and paper or something to make notes with. Detoxing you life is personal and private, so dedicate a notebook to it or open a document on your word processor that no one else has access to, and keep it as your personal property.

This book is designed to help remind you of all the things you can consider that may be relevant in your life. If some aspects of your life are not listed then feel free to include them – you can include absolutely anything that is relevant to you.

When you are analysing different areas of your life you may find that some overlap in a big way. For instance, your friends may also be your work colleagues. In this case, it may be worth assessing them together and separately so that you can look at them in a different light.

Once you have completed the six key tasks, you can then move on to the 25 steps to detoxing your life. Having seen your life in a clearer light, you may decide to do nothing – that is fine. Or you may look at your life and decide that you want to change some aspects of it, in which case these steps should leave you raring to go, and help you to a fully revitalised, and detoxed life.

HOW THIS BOOK WORKS

Detoxing your life is rewarding, refreshing and revitalising but it needs a bit of effort and dedication on your part to get the best results.

All will become crystal clear in the next few pages. But first, here is a simple summary of:

• What you need to do
• What order to do each stage in
• How long each bit should take

Just like an exam paper, you should read the whole section through to check you understand it before you start.

Each stage gets you nearer to knowing exactly what is good for you and what you want, and exactly what is bad for you and what has to go.

1 Compose your mission statement

Give yourself a couple of hours to write your mission statement (see pp. 8 to 16). Then leave it overnight or for a good
period of 'thinking time' and go back to make final changes.
You can always fine-tune your statement but you should
spend time trying to get it right, right from the start.
Knowing what you want in life makes it much easier to get
rid of the stuff you don't want.

2 Complete your own SWOT analysis in each of your six key areas

Give yourself a couple of hours each day to do your SWOT
analysis for each key area (see p. 17). This gives you actual
writing time as well as thinking time in between. Some may
be more relevant to you than others but do them all anyway
and see what they throw up. Once the SWOT is complete,
you will find it easier to decide which bits of your life are
good for you and which bits are definitely bad.

3 Revisit your mission statement

Now you have looked at the finer details of your life, you may
want to make some alterations to your mission statement –
go right ahead.

4 Complete the 25 detox steps

Each step may only take 30 minutes per day to actually do
but will involve a whole lot more thinking and assessment
time. It is probably best to attempt one step per day. This
way, the whole programme will be completed in just over a
month and you will be able to concentrate on how you feel
and what you are thinking. Taking longer will mean that it
starts to interfere with your everyday life too much, whereas

trying to squeeze it into a shorter time will cause you stress and defeat the object – being able to take a good look at what you have, versus what you want.

5 Complete a seven-day dietary detox
This seven-day programme will totally cleanse your insides, and flush out every last toxin from your life.

Writing your mission statement

'The first step to getting somewhere is to decide you don't want to stay where you are.'

Writing your mission statement is very like planning a journey. For instance, you are going to visit some friends who have just moved house. You're not sure how long the journey will take, and you have the whole family in the car. You're certainly going to plan the route or at least look at the map, and make sure you have all the provisions you need. Just knowing their new address won't automatically get you there.

The process of writing your personal mission statement tells you whether you're driving towards your chosen destination or getting hopelessly lost.

Having your own personal mission statement means that you can look at your life and decide if what you are doing is helping you achieve your personal goals, is neutral to achieving your goals, or is actually damaging or working against your goals.

A mission statement tells you WHO YOU ARE and WHO YOU WANT TO BE.

In detox terms, your mission statement is your starting

point for your future. It sets out the main headings under which you put what you want in life and helps you decide what action you need to take.

A good mission statement isn't just a fixed one-liner; it should be broad so that it allows everything in your life to be included.

For example, 'I want to be rich' isn't a good mission statement. It doesn't open many avenues and doesn't inspire you to do much – and it doesn't help you find a way to actually get rich. It doesn't define what 'rich' means to you so how will you know if you are achieving your mission? Do you want to be rich in money terms, rich in happiness or rich in possessions?

Having a more descriptive mission statement will enable you to achieve your mission in a more measurable way. For example, 'I want to create a wealthy life where everything I do is profitable. I want to increase my monetary and my emotional wealth. I can do things that make me happy but earn no money and things that earn money but are not as fulfilling. In this way I can get balance, wealth and happiness.'

This mission statement allows much more flexibility; it is much more specific in some ways but also shows that you are happy to look at different ways to achieve your goals. Some things earn you money and some make you happy. Accepting that you may have to do both to achieve your goals opens up more opportunities, whilst still helping you travel in the right direction.

You have to be very honest with yourself when writing your mission statement. You don't have to go into all the details but you do have to express what you truly want, your own personal mission in life.

Your overall mission is unlikely to change, as it reflects

your true values and beliefs, but the emphasis can vary. It may be predominantly about your career at the moment; it may be about your family; or it may be a bit of everything. But, whatever it is, your actual mission will remain the same – it is your true aim in life.

For example, Deirdre Tox's mission statement might read as follows:

'I want to be successful at work and be the best in my department. I want to get promotion but not to the extent that it interferes with my social life. My friends are very important to me and my current income is enough to enjoy my life as it is. I want to get married eventually and have children when I am ready. I aim to remove all the stress from my life, except for a healthy amount that keeps me on my toes. And I want to save enough money to have at least two weeks holiday abroad every year. If all this has happened at the end of my life then I will have achieved everything I wanted to and more. I will be happy and content.'

Every time Deirdre is considering anything major in her life, or perhaps just something as small as talking to her boss about her job, she can think back to her mission statement and decide whether or not to go ahead, or just be more aware and prepared for the consequences.

For example, being offered a new job that pays a lot of money but means she will be away from home for several weeks at a time may sound interesting; but if what truly makes her happy is having her friends around her then it might not be right to accept it. Alternatively, she could accept the job, knowing that she may feel lonely for a while. But she should then make it a priority to find more friends in her new job.

Knowing your true mission in life helps you to make the

big and small decisions more easily and more effectively, just as knowing your destination helps you look more usefully at the route.

If you don't know where you are headed, then how do you know which direction to go in? And how do you know when you have arrived?

Applying a SWOT analysis

A SWOT analysis is a very useful business tool when planning or assessing a business. When applied personally, it allows you to look at all aspects of your life and then move forward with some key information about what is useful to you and what is not.

SWOT stands for Strengths, Weaknesses, Opportunities and Threats. Applying this analysis to any and every part of your life can very quickly bring to light areas that you need to address. You need to be brutally honest! This 'life' analysis should be private and confidential. Whatever your current situation, to truly detox you need to know all the facts; you need to include everything – good or bad, cruel or kind.

This is what a 'life' SWOT analysis might look like.

What are your strengths?
These are things that you are good at, things that you are happy with. This may change but at this moment in time you find that they support you or give you satisfaction or pleasure. They are things you can build on or use to move forward. For example:

- I enjoy my job
- I can turn my hand to most tasks

- I have a happy, stable relationship and family
- I am creative
- I like to do lots of different things
- I have loads of friends
- I have a mostly good life

What are your weaknesses?

These are things that you don't enjoy or that are bad for you – emotionally or physically. They are things you do or have in your life that you would be better off without, or sorted so that they become strengths.

- I don't like working on stuff I don't like
- I don't like commuting
- I have no best friend to moan with since Sarah moved away
- I feel guilty about leaving the children with the minder while I work
- I want recognition
- I have very little time for just me and my partner without the kids
- I don't like criticism – especially from my new boss
- I find it hard to ask for help
- I need to do lots of different things
- I get bored easily
- I moan a lot

What are your opportunities?

These are things that you might find beneficial or useful if you had some time or determination to actually do them or work on them. They are good things that you just haven't got round to yet!

- I could seek promotion

- I could do some training abroad
- I could introduce new products in my business
- I could find time to introduce new things into my life personally and professionally
- I could have more children
- I could find a new soulmate/best friend

What are your threats?

These are things that you really need to be aware of. Weaknesses are not too damaging because you can generally turn them into strengths with a little time and thought. But threats are things you have to be constantly aware of so that you can stop, remove or prevent them. You need to work on threats sooner rather than later, so you do not suffer their consequences.

- I need to be fitter
- My kids exhaust me
- I have no best friend
- I am losing interest in my job because it's not new any more
- My health seems to be getting worse
- I need vocal support from those around me
- I'm getting bored
- I want change
- I hate my new boss
- I get no support from my bank
- Cash flow is a problem

Once you have completed your SWOT analysis, you have all the pieces of your jigsaw and you can begin to put them together. You have the information to:

- Build on your opportunities
- Strengthen your weaknesses
- Capitalise on your opportunities
- Eliminate or guard against your threats

The mere fact that you have managed to list all these areas means that you have been thinking about your life as a whole – we don't often do that. Now you can see how some aspects of your life affect others and you can look at areas that you need to make some decisions about before they get out of control.

This is your chance to address those problems that you have resigned yourself to living with or put off doing anything about because 'that's just the way it is'.

2

The Detox Your Life Programme – Key Tasks

'There is no going back. Put pen to paper, grey matter into gear and take a good long look at your life.'

To detox your life, you need to:

- Write your mission statement
- Carry out the six key SWOT tasks
- Take the 25 steps to a detoxed life
- Finish with a seven-day dietary detox

The Detox Your Life programme may revolutionise your life or it may just change a few things for the better. It will definitely make you more aware of how you are living now. You can then move forward with the good bits and leave the bad bits behind; or you may decide to deal with the bad bits later on. At least you will know they are there and you can work on them whenever it is the best time for you personally.

THE MISSION STATEMENT

It's time to decide your future – and it is totally up to you . . . Get powerful and decide which direction your life is going in, then start the journey full of energy and excitement.

Now is the time to lay bare your life and all the details that get overlooked or ignored. **It is time to compose your mission statement**.

No one need ever read your mission statement; it can remain totally personal and private. Alternatively, you could make it very public so that everyone knows exactly where you are going – stick it on the fridge door, make a big announcement or simply explain to everyone you know that you have decided to steer your own ship from now on.

The statement can be just one short paragraph or the length of a novel. Whatever it is, it should be what you want for yourself in your life.

This is not a straightforward task and should be treated with respect. Set aside some time in a quiet place so that no one can get hold of you or disturb you. Get a pad and pen, make yourself a drink, switch on the answerphone and collect your thoughts. This is so exciting. From now on, everything you do will benefit you and others instead of just others. Everything you do will move you nearer to your life goals. Even if some things make you take a slight detour, at least you will know how to get back on track. If you choose to do something that has nothing to do with your life mission then that is fine. It means that you are aware of your life and how it is working for you and others, instead of just existing.

Write it now!

Here are some questions you may want to ask yourself to help you along the way:

- What do I want to have done before I die?

- What are the most important issues in my life?

- What job do I want to be doing when I retire?

- Who are the most important people in my life?

- If I could do anything I want with no restrictions, what would it be?

- Am I happy with my health?

- What do I want to change?

- What do I want to keep the same?

THE SWOT ANALYSIS – SIX KEY TASKS

The main areas of your life can be categorised as follows:

- Family
- Friends/social
- Personal relationships
- Work
- Talents/skills/recreation
- Health

Each day you need to carry out a thorough SWOT analysis on one of these areas. This is the toughest but also the most revealing part. Spend at least 30 minutes filling in your SWOT, then revisit it and check that you have thought about absolutely everything that needs to be included. Then think some more – no one said it would be easy!

TASK 1
What are the strengths, weaknesses, opportunities and threats in your *family life*?

Now is the time to write an analysis of your family life.

Your family is where you come from, your roots. Your family need not necessarily be blood related, as many people are adopted or fostered. But, for the purpose of detoxing your life, your family is the group of people who brought you up and the group of people that you bring up – your own children.

Families can be nourishing, nurturing and supportive. They can be fun and sociable and they can be strong and understanding. They can also be nightmares!

You may have thought about starting a family and you may have ideas about how you would like your family to be.

You may doubt your ability to support your family and you may have anxieties about your parenting skills.

If you had a wonderful childhood you may think that you could never recreate this yourself. You therefore begin to doubt your ability to take responsibility for children. This needs thinking about – perhaps you are being a bit tough on yourself?

If you had an unhappy childhood you may desperately want to give your children and family everything they ever want, which may not be a good thing either.

Having a family and being part of a family can be one of the most difficult things in life. We tend to accept our roles because we have no choice. We were born into our family and our children are born to us. There is no choosing; we get what we get.

However, if you do a SWOT analysis on your family life it

may put some issues into perspective. It may also highlight some areas that you think you can change; and it may show you just how good the structure is and how supportive your family can be.

Your SWOT on family life might look something like this:

Strengths
- Social occasions and get-togethers
- Siblings to talk about things with
- Knowledge of family history
- Sense of belonging to a bigger group
- Growing family and satisfaction from watching this
- Unconditional love from parents
- Ready-made friends
- Having children

Weaknesses
- Having to prove self against brothers and sisters
- Having to stay friends even when cross with them
- Too selfish to start own family
- Not having enough time to devote to family
- Easy to think of family last, as they are always there

Opportunities
- Parties at special times of the year
- Having an 'on tap' information source on how to bring up a family
- Having children and sharing everything you have learnt with them
- Babysitting service locally supplied and trustworthy
- Satisfaction of watching children/sisters/brothers/parents grow and change

- Family to tell things to you don't want anyone else to know
- Relatives who have probably experienced everything you are going through

Threats
- Quarrelling
- Not being able to have children
- Children being difficult to deal with
- Not liking every member of family
- Not always liking friends of family

A family SWOT can go on for ever, depending on the extent of your family, if you have children of your own, or even if you are trying for children or thinking about having children. Family SWOTS can be very funny – and also very difficult.

The one sure thing is that your family is there to stay, so it is really useful to see everything about your family situation laid out in front of you. That way, small problems that have been blown out of all proportion can be put into perspective, and larger potential problems can be headed off before they become too difficult to deal with.

If you are thinking about starting a family, there may be many strengths in your situation that you have not considered. Perhaps you have only managed to think through the weaknesses and threats. Alternatively, there may be many more weaknesses and threats than you have managed to think about while getting carried away with dreams of giving birth to several perfect, quiet children who always sleep at the right time.

Getting a balance of strengths, weaknesses, opportunities and threats within your own family is really important because it makes you aware of everything you need to know in order to live with your family for ever and in peace! Surely this alone is reason enough to detox your life . . .

If your family are getting to you then be aware of it and turn to any one of the detox action steps (see Chapter 3) to make you a calmer, more refreshed person who sees every eventuality as a small, easily resolved blip.

TASK 2
What are the strengths, weaknesses, opportunities and threats of your *social life*?

Now is the time to write an analysis of your social life.

If you are ever in a personal relationship and you are treated badly or your partner takes you for granted then people usually advise you to 'finish it before you get hurt'. You tend to be considered foolish if you don't take immediate action.

Yet, if the same is happening with a friendship, we don't seem to follow the same advice. In order to detox your life of unwanted and unproductive relationships you should take the exact same approach with so-called friends. Carrying out a SWOT of your friends will help you decide if the friend who has always caused you problems or heartache should now become simply an acquaintance.

Good friends can help you through the most wonderful and the most terrible of times. You can build a relationship with a good friend that, with very little effort, can provide all the support you ever need in your life: someone to be happy with, someone to cry with, someone to shop with, someone to do absolutely nothing with, someone to complain to and someone to 'be the first to know'. If you have good friends and are a good friend yourself, you need little else.

Then there are friends who don't do any of the above: friends who just seem to drain you and always take without replenishing. We can all take from our friends but if this isn't eventually balanced by letting them take from us then the relationship becomes uneven and one-sided. It is no longer beneficial to both parties, only one; and it can actually become detrimental to your health and your happiness.

These types of friends have to go. Or at least you have to be aware of what they can do to you; and you need to protect yourself from the downside so that you can concentrate on the beneficial side of the relationship.

Doing a SWOT on your social life can be difficult; simply putting friends' names into the categories of Strengths, Weaknesses, Opportunities and Threats doesn't work. To really analyse your friends and social life you need to do a SWOT on what you need from friends and acquaintances, what you give and take from people you know, and then see who can deliver against your criteria and who doesn't fit into any of the categories.

It is also good to plan the SWOT out because it will demonstrate to you the type of friend you are and what types of friends you have. Then you can make a decision to keep things the same or to change the bits you are not quite so keen on.

Strengths
- Being there when something goes wrong
- Offering unconditional friendship
- Enjoying lots of company
- Quite positive
- Willing to help out

- Quite broad-minded
- Not easily shocked

Weaknesses
- Don't take criticism easily
- Don't like cancellations
- Talk about self a lot
- Always try to find experience with which to compare
- Want to be popular
- Saying yes to helping everyone all the time
- Spending time with X but not really liking her

Opportunities
- Can make friends easily
- Learn to take criticism
- Listen more

Threats
- Tend to decide if like or dislike on only a moment's meeting
- Don't like meeting new people much
- Don't always trust instincts

Once you have completed your own personal friendship SWOT, you can begin to see how your friends fill your needs and how you fill theirs. It may become clear that there are some people in your life who just don't seem to fit in at any point and whose names you cannot put against any of your SWOT. They drain you mentally, and constantly drone on about themselves.

It is now time to consider how to move forward. Maybe a friend or acquaintance does so much harm and puts you down so much that you decide never to call them again. If such a relationship peters out it is a positive thing – you have cleared out a negative person from your life.

Or you may decide that you should see some of your friends much more often because you get a real buzz from being with them. They may not seem to be the best 'match' for you as a friend, but perhaps they counter your bad points, so you can improve by spending more time enjoying each other's company.

There may be other friends who are perfect matches for you. Be aware of this and see how you can nurture each other. If they are good listeners, talk with them more and see where it leads.

Having done the SWOT, you may have a friend who positively drives you bananas and now you can see why – they are probably the direct opposite of you in what they bring to a relationship. This is a great finding and can help you understand the special relationship you have. You will never change each other but this unusual friendship will make much more sense from now on.

Don't keep a friendship that upsets you or damages you – that is not a friendship. There are plenty of people you need to deal with on a day-to-day basis who you don't like or wouldn't choose to have as a friend. So take the opportunity, if you have it, to change the situation and spend less and less time with someone who doesn't make your life better and more positive.

TASK 3
What are the strengths, weaknesses, opportunities and threats in your *personal life*?

Now is the time to write an analysis of your personal life.

The SWOT analysis of your personal life will actually look remarkably similar to your friendship SWOT. The qualities required in a friendship are the same as those in a relationship because friendship is one of the most important elements of a partnership.

If your personal relationship is going well, you will probably feel that you do not need to complete the SWOT in this section. But do it anyway because there may be improvements you can make or new discoveries that come to light. You may find that you can contribute more to the relationship. Don't always see SWOT analysis from your point of view – see it from the other person's point of view too. You may gain some surprising insights . . .

Relationships are brilliant when they are going well – they can feel fulfilling, invigorating, refreshing, pleasing, wonderful, freeing, educational and much, much more. When they aren't going well, relationships are awful. They drain, they frustrate, they upset, they anger, they empty, and they are plainly bad for your health.

We stay in bad relationships longer than we need to. We wait for something to change and start to get better without making much effort, or we make loads of effort and there is still no change.

If you take the time to look at your relationship properly, you should be in a position to decide whether or not to finish it, or whether to move it on to the next stage.

First you need to know what you want out of a relationship. If you don't know that, how can you possibly know if it is going well or not?

Doing a SWOT on your personal life doesn't mean drawing up a wish list for your ideal partner but it will make you aware of how a very important part of your life is going. It is not an excuse to run away when things are not going according to plan but it does give you the chance to see what is happening, to decide whether or not you are happy with the situation, and what, if anything, you should do about it.

Strengths
- I love my partner
- I am loved back
- We are a team
- We go to lots of places together
- I can see that we have a future
- I like doing things together
- We are stronger together than apart

Weaknesses
- We don't make as much time for our friends
- We don't enjoy the same hobbies
- We enjoy different sorts of foods
- I nag too much
- I end up doing lots of housework

Opportunities
- We could do lots more together
- We could spend the rest of our lives together
- We could develop some shared interests

- I could learn from my partner
- I could use my partner for support and help
- My partner could help give me confidence

Threats
- Taking each other for granted
- Not making the effort when we should
- Getting into a rut
- Not surprising each other
- Not calling each other for a chat
- Not sharing everyday situations or problems
- Not giving each other space
- Not making sure we share quality time

After completing your SWOT you should find things that both of you can do to improve your personal relationship. If you only find that there are things your partner should be doing for you then you should revisit the threats section and put in there that you are always right. This is a threat because if you believe it you are probably fooling yourself. And if you are not fooling yourself, maybe there are some areas you have forgotten to include.

There may be some things that will improve the balance in every area of your relationship and there may well be things that you need to give special attention to in order to save the relationship. You may want to open this section up to your partner. Get them to complete their own SWOT and then you can make the time to sit and go through the results together. You never know – perhaps there are things you do without thinking that drive your partner wild with happiness and other things that drive them mad with frustration.

Meet those festering problems head on and deal with them before they get the chance to become an issue.

Get personal and detox your relationship.

TASK 4
What are the strengths, weaknesses, opportunities and threats in your *work life*?

Now is the time to write an analysis of your working life.

You spend approximately 24 per cent of your life working, which sounds as if you have over 75 per cent of your life to do just what you want . . . This is not quite true.

On average we:
- Sleep for 33 per cent (eight hours per night)
- Enjoy weekends for 28 per cent (104 days per year)
- Have 15 per cent free time

So, working for 24 per cent of your life begins to sound like quite a lot of time. And that estimate doesn't even take over-time into consideration, or the work you take home or the time you spend thinking about work.

In short, your job is really very important to your quality of life. So, are you doing a job you want to do? Is it giving you the returns you want or is it giving you grief?

With a little planning and thought, and perhaps a little training, you may be able to make changes to your job that make your life infinitely better. So do your SWOT.

Strengths
- Good with people
- Good at teamwork

- Good at getting in early
- Good at socialising
- Good at customer relations
- Good at marketing

Weaknesses

- Can't do the hard sell
- Don't like criticism
- Take criticism personally
- Get bored easily
- Don't think about the figures
- Don't like targets
- Don't like working weekends or overtime

Opportunities

- Will travel a bit
- Will learn, go on courses, etc
- Want promotion
- Want more responsibility to allay boredom
- Have car
- Can work from home

Threats

- Bit lazy if bored
- Need encouragement to motivate
- Need to feel loved to feel happy
- Feel isolated if working alone
- Feel the need to 'play to an audience'
- Don't work well on own
- Can't restrict spending

Once you have written down your SWOT analysis, you can

see if your current job is fulfilling your needs now. Can you develop into areas that hold potential for you? Or are you in a 'dead end' job that will only ever fulfil some of your needs?

Changing jobs is not that easy. But, again, you can only make the decision to go for another job if you take the time to look at what you have now. Job satisfaction can really change your life. Just knowing what you get from your job and what you can give to this 24 per cent of your life can make a big difference to your frame of mind.

TASK 5
What are the strengths, weaknesses, opportunities and threats of your *recreational life*?

Now is the time to write an analysis of your recreational life.

We decide what we are good at when we are at school. It doesn't matter that we may have developed skills since then or inadvertently found something that we like doing and are good at. We still 'know' what we can and cannot do. School has a lot going for it but if you believe your education taught you everything you will ever know, think again! In fact, it taught you the basics; it planted the seeds for you to grow. If you think about it there are many things they could not possibly teach you at school, but they *did* prepare you for a great deal of future learning.

There are many things you do in your life for enjoyment that could be increased or reintroduced. Think about all the things that you are now an expert in and enjoy doing but have never really looked at it in that way. For instance:

- How could you possibly learn about having a family?

- How great are you at taking a picnic to the park to just chill out and catch up?

- How could you possibly know you would be great at staying calm when the central heating has failed on a frosty morning?

- How could they have taught you about getting from one end of the country to the other?

- Remember you love simply swimming in a pool for relaxation.

- Who taught you to seek out all the own-brand labels when you are on a tight budget?

- No one taught you to mediate between friends who are arguing about who left the top off the toothpaste.

- Think how good you feel after a long country walk.

- You forget that you are an expert at just listening.

- You are now a graduate in expressing your feelings and getting things sorted before they cause real damage . . .

If you think about it you have some of the most brilliant skills available to man. And you thought that a few qualifications on a strip of paper represented all that you were good at!

Do a SWOT analysis right now. I bet the only threat you find will be a little bit of disbelief about the fact that you have discovered you are the world's greatest person at nearly everything you do.

Once you have completed your list, look at it and decide if

there is anything you want to develop in your new-found skills.

So do your SWOT.

Strengths
- Love reading
- Like being outdoors
- Can get friends together quickly
- Love being with family for days out

Weaknesses
- Find maths hard
- Don't like strenuous exercise
- Sometimes need outside motivation
- Can get stuck in a rut

Opportunities
- Have lots of time on Sundays to do things
- Have an open mind most of the time

Threats
- Don't have much spare cash
- Spare time often gets used up at work
- Friends are unable to find time to spend together

TASK 6

What are the strengths, weaknesses, opportunities and threats of your *health*?

Now is the time to write an analysis of your health.

Getting rid of unhealthiness and unfitness is a more motivating way of looking at getting fit and healthy. 'Getting fit and healthy' sounds like we have to actively change everything about our lives and become something that is not natural to us. Yet, if we flip the coin and realise that we are by nature fit and healthy and that it is us that do things to make ourselves unhealthy, then all we need to do is eliminate these things and we will become healthy naturally!

Looking at your health is also important when detoxing your life, as it can often mean the difference between success and failure. If you are feeling good and healthy then you have the strength and stamina to sort your problems out and make the best of all the good times. But if you are exhausted and feeling ill then it is really hard to deal with anything – good or bad. Simply wanting to curl up and go to sleep for a week is not the best way to feel detoxed and liberated.

If you are intending to fully detox yourself there are plenty of books available that can take you through the process step by step (e.g. my book *Detox Yourself*). But even if you don't want to do a full-scale detox, you can still make some major changes in your health with a few simple tweaks.

The first thing is to do your SWOT analysis. Write down everything you do that affects your physical health, diet and fitness.

Strengths
- Like fresh fruit and vegetables
- Like drinking water
- Like exercise when I get into it
- Like glowing skin
- Like sleeping well
- Like having lots of energy

Weaknesses
- Takes a long time to get into exercise
- Like coffee every day (four or five cups)
- Like wine (share a bottle every Friday/Saturday/Sunday)
- Like eating out (about three evenings per week plus take-aways)
- Love chips and bacon sandwiches
- Often eat late at night and go straight to bed

Opportunities
- Get into exercise
- Am a member of a gym
- Can get aromatherapy at discount price

Threats
- Get tired – not enough sleep
- Can get very lazy if not motivated
- Can eat junk food – especially in winter
- Can drink too much caffeine very easily
- Get spotty if too much alcohol
- Weight gain

Now, look at your analysis and see how you can use all the categories to your advantage. Then start to formulate your physical health flow chart. Include all the things you do that are positive and all the things you do that are negative. (You are definitely allowed some negatives – it is just that you need to make sure they are balanced or outweighed by positives.)

Your weekly health flow chart might look something like this:

Positives

- Eat fruit every day
- Eat vegetables every day
- Take exercise every other day for 40 minutes
- Facial every month (home-made or professional)
- Treatment every two months e.g. massage, aromatherapy, reflexology etc.
- Drink 3 pints of water every day (one glass per hour)
- Two days per week on preservative-free food
- Eat before 8pm five nights a week and never later than 9pm
- Go to bed before 11pm five nights a week

Negatives

- Seven glasses of wine a week (never more than two in any one sitting!)
- One bacon sandwich per week (enjoy it, instead of four per week without thinking)
- One portion of chips per week
- One proper coffee per day
- Three exercise-free days per week
- Two late nights a week

By making a few rules, you can still do some bad things while ultimately improving your health.

3.

25 Steps to a Fully Detoxed Life

Most of the hard work has been done – now the fun starts.

The next 25 days are full of ways to clear the clutter, even out the excess, and pare down to the place you want to be.

You have just spent time looking at and assessing the bigger issues in your life. (Keep reflecting on your mission statement and SWOT analysis to check whether you are keeping your life on track.)

Now is the time to detox the details – the details that you probably don't think about or are not even aware of. Changing small details makes it easier to change big issues, chipping away until you are left with everything you want and nothing that you don't want.

Each of the 25 steps is designed to change your life in some way or another. Some will be just one-off exercises for you to do and see how they change things, and some steps will be new things to include in your life from this point onwards.

I recommend that you try to take a day to do each of the 25 steps. Take a break every now and then but try to keep it within a month. This way, you can add to and change your life gradually. Take a day here and there to just see the differences in your life and a day here and there to reflect on how well you are doing, then go on to the next step.

It may sound easy but you need to realise that you are changing or reassessing the habits of a lifetime. You will be learning new things to do and new things to say – 'I want', 'No thank you' and 'I need help' are all examples of new phrases that you will be using. The next few days will make you braver and more appreciative of yourself.

If you detox the small stuff, then the bigger stuff takes care of itself. Together with your new-found knowledge of what you do and don't want in your life, you will emerge a new and vibrant person – on your own personal mission.

You just get to do exactly what you want to from now on.

STEP 1
Detox your life of chemical stimulants

Start by purging the manufactured stimulants from your life and see how it feels to gain energy with no toxic waste or side effects. Let your body do what it is naturally designed to do and feel the benefits.

This step is designed to get you into the habit of allowing your body to produce its own natural stimulants instead of relying on artificial ones. Once you have made these changes, you should stick with them. Step 1 is a change for life.

Our bodies are very clever. We know this because cavemen survived quite happily without the use of chocolate munchies and vitamin supplements.

If there is something lacking in our diet we get ill or show symptoms. We then take the necessary action and rectify any problems – our bodies have told us what we need.

Nowadays – because we are so developed and ingenious – we have started to invent and develop alternatives to the natural solutions.

For instance, if we feel tired we drink coffee, but our bodies are asking for sleep. If we are thirsty we drink pints of beer, but our bodies are asking for water. If we feel weak we take vitamins and carry on eating snack food, but our bodies are asking for a balanced diet.

Our bodies try to adapt and use these substitutes as effectively as possible. Soon we see the chemical/manufactured alternative as the only solution. But using powerful artificial stimulants can result in anxiety, high blood pressure and insomnia, or restless and fitful sleep.

This is because using artificial stimulants results in an immediate rise in blood sugar and a preparation of the adrenal glands – the 'high'. Once this occurs, we are prepared to expend physical and mental energy. But we don't use it. We simply carry on doing what we do, and so we have an immediate crash of energy which is often called the 'low'. What do we do when we are low? Create another high – with more caffeine, more sugar, more alcohol. And so the cycle continues.

This continuous roller-coaster of chemical highs and lows will eventually lead to dependency. More than two portions or drinks of any given artificial stimulant a day will cause your body to adapt to the stimulant's availability. Coming off it is likely to cause headaches, tiredness and general lethargy.

Depending on how much you have used chemical stimulants, your 'withdrawal' symptoms may last for up to several days. A mild headache is hopefully the worst you will experience but only you will know how dependent you have been on these substances.

Coffee, tea, sugar and alcohol are the most commonly used artificial stimulants. Cutting these out should ideally be done gradually, over a period of a few weeks, but you may decide to do it overnight.

Once you have cut these out of your life, or drastically cut down to using an artificial stimulant only once a day, your body will begin to realise that the chemical version is not available and will start to produce the relevant stimulants naturally and in the doses required. Removing the highs and lows will make your moods more even, your energy levels more balanced, and your daily life more peaceful. You should sleep more soundly and your skin will look wonderful, as you are no longer pumping your body full of chemicals.

Carry out the following self-assessment, take the necessary action and detox all dangerous chemical stimulants from your life.

Stimulant assessment

I currently drink:

1–2 cups of coffee and/or tea per day (caffeinated or decaffeinated)	1
3–5 cups of coffee and/or tea per day (caffeinated or decaffeinated)	2
more than 6 cups of coffee and/or tea per day (caffeinated or decaffeinated)	3

I currently snack on:

1 or less bars of chocolate per day	1
2 or more sugary snacks per day	2

I currently drink:

1–2 measures* of alcohol per day	1
3–4 measures of alcohol per day	2
4 or more measures of alcohol per day	3

(*1 measure = 1 glass of wine, 1 measure of spirits or 1 pint of beer)

If you score more than 3 points then you should definitely cut down on the stimulants you are using.

Natural stimulants cost nothing and are readily available. Get some balance in your life, detox the chemicals and feel the natural high.

STEP 2
Detox your immune system

Banish illness and never 'feel under the weather' again by boosting your immune system. Any germ daring to enter your body will immediately be blasted and destroyed, leaving you to get on with more worthwhile things. A little effort each day, from now on, could bring huge benefits in the future.

Many of us seem to be getting more colds and illnesses. They hang on for much longer and then we catch something else because our immune systems have been weakened, due to the fact that they have just been fighting an illness . . . And so the loop continues.

If you are repeatedly getting ill or feeling under the weather then it may be that you never really let your body get

back to full fitness after a previous illness. This can be dangerous and may also lead you to accept feeling 'below par' as the
norm.

There are many things you can do to boost and strengthen
your body's immunity. You may not wish to do them all. But
you can select from them to form your own regime that will
let you take charge of your own health. Taking the following
steps will give your body a great chance to be fit, healthy and
full of vitality.

- Drink loads of water (up to 3 pints or 1.5 litres is the norm
  for a normally active adult). If you have a specially active
  job or life then you must increase these amounts. Drink
  over the whole day and do not have too much liquid in the
  evening, as this may disrupt your sleep.

- Include as many types as possible of fresh fruits, vegetables,
  meats and fish in your diet. A balanced diet will ensure a
  good spread of nutrients, vitamins and minerals and
  changing proteins is reported to keep the immune system
  more alert.

- Use natural remedies to boost your immune system and
  help fight infection.

You may already know of some supplements you can take but
here is a selection. Take a look and think about including one
or some of them in your day-to-day detox regime to boost
your immune system.

In all cases you should read the dosage details on the pack-
aging before taking any. It is always better to take a few
high-quality products that answer your personal needs, rather
than taking a bit of everything and never knowing what is
having an effect.

A few carefully chosen supplements, together with increased water intake, and a high-quality, varied diet should detox and clean you out, leaving you ready to face anything the world can throw at you.

Acidophilus supplements
Your body is full of friendly bacteria – *Lactobacillus acidophilus* – designed to keep you in perfect balance but antibiotics can destroy it. When this friendly bacteria is under threat, or has been invaded by enemy bacteria, taking an acidophilus supplement will help you keep the tox out of your system. It will synthesise B vitamins and help to fight off enemy bacteria (such as salmonella, candida (thrush) and many more). Acidophilus should be stored in the fridge and taken with mineral water, as directed on the bottle.

Vitamin C
Regular vitamin C supplements have been recommended for many years, and this is based on sound research. Vitamin C strengthens the blood vessels and helps the body fight infection. Taken regularly, it should reduce the effects of the cold germ and prevent the body developing allergies. It should also help to build strong bones.

Echinacea
Echinacea is a Native American herb which has increased in popularity in recent years. Many people take it on a regular basis to prevent colds and flu taking hold. It is also said to be anti-ageing, due to its immune-enhancing and antibiotic properties. Take 15 drops in water a couple of times a day and you should never fall prey to the common cold again.

Garlic

Garlic will ward off germs as well as vampires! It will increase your circulation, so you can wave goodbye to red noses and cold toes, while boosting your immune system. Ideally, one raw clove a day will keep harm at bay but this can be a little anti-social; an odourless perle or tablet each day can be equally effective.

Ginko biloba

Ginko biloba also increases blood circulation and is said to improve brain power too, so get healthy and wise at the same time.

Tea tree oil

Fantastically popular with our antipodean friends, tea tree oil is an all-round top performer in the anti-fungal/antiseptic field. Dab on spots for rapid relief. Alternatively, bathe feet in a bowl including a few drops of the tincture and watch any fungal infection clear before your very eyes.

Milk thistle

Although not an excuse to over-indulge, milk thistle is fantastic for detoxing your liver so it is fast becoming the cure for the morning after! There are also claims that it contains elements that stimulate growth of liver cells.

Remember, a regular multivitamin, mineral or herbal supplement can help fill any gaps in your diet whilst you change from an unhealthy to a healthy one. But don't use supplements as substitutes for a good, varied diet.

You can also take supplements to stop germs getting to you quite so readily, although there's no need to become obsessive. These are purely sensible everyday measures to keep the tox out of your life.

Don't ignore the very sensible advice we all had drilled into us as children. Wash your hands when dealing with food, between dealing with cooked and raw food and always after visiting the toilet.

Drip-dry your hands. Don't wipe them on your clothes, as they probably carry loads of old germs. Alternatively, use hot air dryers or paper towels – not tea towels!

Throw away kitchen cloths regularly and clean all cutting boards, using separate boards for raw and cooked foods.

Don't worry too much ... We are designed to fight infection but there are some small things we can do to enable our bodies to become so much more efficient at doing so.

Cold? What cold!

STEP 3
Breathe for life

Proper, deep breathing reduces stress, improves immunity and boosts energy levels. It will detox your life of tension and introduce pure calm and relaxation.

Everyone knows how important oxygen is for our survival but they are much less sure of how to breathe correctly or what effects good breathing has.

We know that even a momentary lack of the correct level of oxygen in the body can result in serious damage or even death. Yet many of us continue to underuse our lungs and deprive our bodies of all the benefits of correct breathing.

From early childhood we are told to 'stand up straight,

stomachs in'. When we are told to take a deep breath we automatically inhale and raise our chest. But, by restricting movement of the stomach and abdomen, we are limiting the area that our lungs can expand into. We therefore develop the habit of only using a third of our lung capacity each time we inhale.

The balance of your mind and body is also affected by your breathing. If you are tense and stressed, and your breathing is short and shallow, you are less likely to be able to think straight, your movements become erratic and your balance is thrown. Yet correct breathing is easy and much more relaxing.

To breathe correctly, you simply relax your stomach muscles, inhale through your nose slowly and take in the air until it feels as if the base of your stomach is full of it. Pause momentarily and then exhale through the mouth. When you feel the air 'in your stomach' it shows that you have relaxed your diaphragm muscle, which means your lungs have fully expanded and you have inhaled to full capacity. This will feel strange at first but will soon become such a normal way to breathe you won't need to think about it any more.

Deeper breathing slows the heart rate and the pulse. The deeper we breathe, the more oxygen we inhale. All these are indications of improved and stronger health.

A simple breathing exercise

This is a good breathing exercise to do when you feel stressed, if you cannot sleep or if you simply want to recharge your batteries:

- Sit comfortably or lie down, supporting your lower back with a cushion if necessary.

- Place your hands on your stomach area, with the fingertips just touching.

- Start to breathe in through your nose very slowly, to the count of four. (As you inhale, you should feel your stomach expand and your fingertips separate.)

- Hold the breath for four and exhale slowly through your mouth, to a count of eight.

- Repeat several times as required.

It will feel strange at first, as you are not used to using your muscles to expand your stomach in this way, but over a period of just a few minutes this will become more natural.

Continue this exercise for at least ten inward breaths and you should feel much more relaxed and 'centred'. Eventually you will not need to use your fingers to check that your stomach is expanding (rather than your chest). Soon you will be able to carry out the exercise whilst you are going about your normal day-to-day business – not the lying down but the controlled breathing! If you ever have difficulty dropping off to sleep, this is a far more effective way than the traditional 'counting sheep'. The chances are that you won't make it to ten – you will probably be asleep by six.

We live by our breathing so learn to do it properly and live a little bit more.

STEP 4
Detox your mind

Positive thinking improves your everyday quality of life – suddenly nothing seems so difficult any more.

Mental fitness is just as important as physical fitness. Positive thinking, self-esteem and mental agility are vital to keeping yourself detoxed of negative feelings. Instead of getting trapped in a downward spiral you can learn how to turn any negative into a huge positive.

If you know what you want in life and how to go about getting it, everything you do will be to your advantage. If you know how to clear out the stuff that gets in the way of your true goals, you will have more space to think about yourself. Thinking about yourself isn't selfish, because if you are happy and contented with your thoughts then you can pass that happiness and contentment on to others. Laughter is catching, and so is moaning, and we all know which one we would prefer to catch.

If everyone knew more about themselves, and what they wanted in life, the world would be a great place, because everyone would help each other out just by getting on with it.

Start doing the following five exercises every day and see how good it feels:

1. Write a list

Before you go to sleep each night, write a list of things you need to do tomorrow, in order of priority.

Writing a list will help you sleep better at night because you will have relieved your mind of the 'I must remember to . . .' pressure. You will also be able to prioritise your most important tasks and you will feel satisfied once you have completed them and 'crossed them off your list' (literally).

2. Smile

Smile at everything that deserves a smile and see how many times your smile is returned.

Smiling makes you feel good – it can make a bad or unhappy situation into a good or happy one.

3. Take a break and 'smell the roses'

Be aware of everything around you for the next hour. Don't just walk past the flowers thinking they probably smell nice – actually stop and enjoy the fragrance. Don't just look at the view and think you have seen it a thousand times – actually look at it and see what has changed and what is good. Don't chew your food and think of your next meeting – actually chew the food and enjoy the taste and texture. Is it crunchy, is it sweet, is it soft or is it spicy? Chew the food and taste the difference.

4. Tell someone you think they are great

You probably often think that people around you are good at something, look particularly well, that their perfume smells nice or they have been really helpful. Well, say it to them. Tell them they look good, tell them they have been helpful, tell them you think they are good at something.

Everyone knows how nice it feels to get a compliment so make someone's day and let them know what you are thinking. It feels just as good to give a compliment as it does to receive one.

5. Change a negative into a positive

Whenever anything goes wrong or is annoying, find three ways to make it positive.

For instance, I miss the bus and will be late for work:

1. I will call the office and tell them when I expect to get in so no one wonders where I am.

2. I will go to the supermarket until the next bus is due.

3. I will cook a lovely meal with the food I bought and invite a friend for an impromptu evening.

I catch the next bus and feel good.

You see – three steps to change a bad into a good.

Happiness and positive thinking bring personal success and personal success brings happiness. Get some peace and contentment – detox your mind.

STEP 5
Feed your brain

A clear, crisp mind can see the solutions laid out before it. A clear, crisp mind will sort the waste and detox the fuzziness; it will hone in on the relevant and get you where you want to be, with no wasteful detours. Eat your way to intelligence and chomp your way to cheeriness.

It should come as no surprise that the sorts of foods that

are good for your brain, intelligence, memory, alertness and vitality are also the types of foods that are good for you in all sorts of other ways.

Following a balanced diet will provide all the nutrients you need to keep your mind alert and fit for the Detox Your Life tasks, so you don't miss anything important.

'Balanced' is the key word – we should cut down on some foods and increase others in order to fulfil all our nutritional requirements.

We should also watch what we eat and when in order to ensure optimum energy levels at the times we most require them. Everyone has suffered the mid-afternoon 'snooze' syndrome where we are expected to carry on with the day as normal when all we really want to do is sit in a big comfortable chair and have a nice sleep for half an hour. Maintaining a continuous level of blood sugar is vital if we want to avoid these 'dips' of energy and brain function during the day.

For this reason, three meals a day may not be the ultimate way to nourish our bodies. Eating a large breakfast, lunch and evening meal will lead to a blood sugar low before each of these meals, as the body has used all its energy. A blood sugar high will then occur directly after eating – which always results in a low an hour or so later, depending on the content of each meal. If the carbohydrates consumed are carefully chosen then the major peaks and troughs can be avoided but often this is not the case.

During the Detox Your Life programme you should try to eat five or six smaller meals during the day in order to ensure the continuous levels of alertness required to fulfil your tasks.

You should limit (or, ideally, eliminate) some foods during the programme as these are likely to inhibit correct absorption of some essential nutrients – you don't want anything to stop you from getting the best out of all your hard work.

The best way to achieve optimum nutrition is to change your current eating regime to incorporate the required nutrients – simply taking supplements is a lazy way to change your diet and we really *are* what we eat.

'Everything in moderation' is a very good approach when it comes to food. Our bodies respond badly when we over-indulge in anything.

Here are some other tips that will help you keep mentally alert throughout your life-changing programme:

- Eat regular, small meals. Five or six small meals eaten regularly will keep you more mentally alert than two or three big meals.

- Eat breakfast. Low blood sugar in the morning adversely affects your memory and ability to concentrate. Breakfast will wake your brain. If you try to work without first eating a small breakfast then your body is likely to ask for short-term chemical stimulants – coffee, tea, sugar, chocolate, etc. If you have breakfast then you will satisfy your energy needs and your body can operate efficiently.

- Eat a mid-morning snack consisting of a slow-release carbohydrate such as wholemeal bread or oatcakes. (These are foods that release energy steadily over a longer period of time avoiding the energy surges and dips that come with sugary or refined foods like biscuits, cakes and white bread.) A slow-release snack will stave off any hunger pangs and keep energy at a constant level.

- Eat lunch as normal but make it light and refreshing, including lots of fresh, raw vegetables.

- Eat a mid-afternoon snack to prevent the 'snooze' require-ment. Again, a healthy, low-refined sugar, slow-release energy food will make sure you don't create any problem-atic highs and lows – fruit such as bananas, apples and pears are great for this.

- Supper in the evening should be kept healthy and not necessarily the largest meal of the day – equal portions for breakfast, lunch and evening meal will help keep your brain working efficiently, and the snacks should be lighter.

- A final snack before bed is fine but make sure it doesn't contain anything that will prevent you from getting a good night's sleep. If you know your own culprits, fine but gener-ally avoid stimulants like chocolate, cheese and caffeine.

- You should have your meals and snacks at roughly equal intervals. For example, if your day starts at 8am, you could have your meals as follows:

  8.30   Breakfast
  11.00   Mid-morning snack
  1.30   Lunch
  3.30   Light snack
  6.30   Supper
  9.30   Light snack

- If you have ever suspected that you may be intolerant of foods such as wheat or dairy products, this is the ideal opportunity to exclude them from your diet to see if you feel different as a result.

- Try to keep the foods as natural as possible (e.g. whole grains rather than refined) and try to cook them as little as possible. Obviously, fish and meat should be thoroughly cooked (unless you convert to eating lots of Japanese raw fish which would be great for the programme). Vegetables should be a balance of raw, lightly stir-fried or quickly grilled to keep all the nutrients in them. Fruit is easy to eat raw and you should eat at least five pieces a day. Pasta, rice, bread and potatoes, grains, pulses, etc should be cooked as directed but always so that you give your jaw a good workout. This means the goodness has not been completely boiled away and that you will get great muscle tone in your face from chewing them!

• Most stimulants and chemicals should be out of your life by now but here's a full list, just in case any culprits have slipped through the net:

Caffeine: Limit your intake of any caffeine product (tea, coffee, cola, chocolate) to one per day – or cut them out altogether.

Alcohol: Limit your intake of alcohol to one unit per day – these units may not be 'saved'. One or no units per day is the maximum permitted.

Sugary products: Cakes, biscuits, crisps, sweets, chocolate bars and all things 'naughty' should be eliminated or limited to one *small* slice/piece/packet/bar per day. These foods are high in calories and sugars – they will give you a boost but it will be swiftly followed by a drowsy 'low'.

Fats: Products high in saturated fats (e.g. meat and cheese) should be avoided. Fat intake should be limited to polyunsaturates, oily fish, nuts and oils.

Smoking/Pollution: Airborne pollution and smoking – passive or active – should be avoided at all costs. If you smoke then give up now! And if you can avoid spending time in public areas that smokers use or outside areas that have heavy traffic then do. Smoking and pollution not only have the obvious side effects of nicotine/passive smoking/addiction, but they also prevent complete absorption of vitamins and minerals from foods, they dull your tastebuds and damage skin tone, complexion and general health.

There are some specific nutrients that are reputed to have very definite effects on our brains. I have listed these below, with their natural food sources. It is much better to incorporate these foods in your diet, so that your body can assimilate them naturally, than to take expensive supplements and pills.

Nutrient	Role	Food sources
Choline	Aids memory	Vegetables, egg yolks
DMAE*	Elevates mood, improves memory and increases intelligence	Fish, especially anchovies and sardines
Inositol	Nourishes brain cells	Grapefruit, cabbage
Niacin	Maintains healthy nervous system and brain function	Liver, kidney, fish, eggs, poultry, avocado, peaches
Sulphur	Maintains oxygen balance for brain function	Fish, eggs, cabbage
Zinc	Improves brain function and mental alertness	Wheatgerm, pumpkin seeds, eggs, ground mustard
Tryptophan	Essential amino acid – for brain to produce serotonin	Milk, fish, turkey, bananas, dried dates, peanuts

*dimethylaminoethanol

Phenylalanine	Essential amino acid – to improve memory and mental alertness	Protein-rich foods, soy products, almonds, pumpkin and sesame seeds
Carbohydrates	Provides essential energy for brain and central nervous system	Bread, pasta, pulses, rice, oats, potatoes and sweet potatoes
Iodine	Improves readiness and pace of brain	Kelp, onions and sea-food

(Information taken from *The Vitamin Bible*, Earl Mindell, Arlington Books; and *The Optimum Nutrition Bible*, Patrick Holford, Piatkus Books.)

A balanced diet will give you all these nutrients, in the correct form. Taking supplements of these vitamins and minerals is not recommended unless you have first consulted a nutritionist or your doctor. You may also wish to see a nutritionist if you are currently taking any prescribed drugs or the contraceptive pill, as many medicines can prevent the body from absorbing essential nutrients or can deplete the body's natural stores.

Having said that you should incorporate all these nutrients in their natural food forms, it is not always easy to include so many foodstuffs in your daily diet. See Chapter 5 for some recipes that will make sure you stay full of energy and get your fill of 'brain foods'.

Start the day with stimulating energy food. Juicing, either by using a juice extractor or by simply peeling fruit and putting delicious combinations in a liquidiser, is great, and fruit is a must at breakfast. It is also good to have some protein (e.g. milk or yoghurt) to keep your energy levels up until lunchtime.

Try the delicious brain-feeding recipes in Chapter 5 and cook your way to a cleaner, cleverer you!

STEP 6
Work with the seasons

Nature intends things to grow at certain times of the year. Sticking to eating what's in season means we eat what nature intends, when and how nature intends it – quite naturally. Detox the forcing, processing and storing, and keep to freshly picked produce, full of vitality.

Wild plants seed, grow, flower and die in rotation. The weather grows cold, freezes, warms up, becomes hot and then cools down again. The planets move around, giving us seasons, tides, day and night, dark and light. All this happens continuously and without any help from us.

If we truly ate according to the seasons, we would have hearty vegetables and pulses in the winter months, fresh crispy vegetables and fruits in the spring, delicate light vegetables and succulent perfumed fruits in the summer, and finally deep red and russet fruits and vegetables in the autumn.

Everything has a time and every time has a season. We have illnesses associated with seasons. We get colds in winter, hayfever in summer.

Some people try to change this rhythm by going away on holiday to a foreign country, or by eating foods from a different season, or by having treatment for illnesses such as SAD (Seasonal Affective Disorder), using artificial light to bring spring into winter.

Despite everything being natural and happening naturally we seem to be addicted to trying to change it.

We fly foods in from around the world so that we can have them all year round. We expect to be able to buy every kind of flower all year round. We complain in the winter that it is too cold and then we moan in the summer that it is too hot. If it rains after a long, dangerous drought it is miserable, despite the fact that we have been rescued from hosepipe bans and water rationing. We put an awful lot of energy and thought into something that we just cannot change!

To list absolutely everything that is 'in season' would fill a book itself but there are some helpful pointers to finding out what you should be eating and when.

For instance, colour is a good way of thinking through the seasons. We already have colours that we associate with the seasons and use terms like 'spring feel', 'warm autumn tones', 'dark wintery' and 'bright summery' colours. If in doubt, you can keep these colours in mind when shopping and you should be able to make a fair guess.

Spring is the season of growth, a time of lambing, a time to sow seed early and see it sprout in late spring. Spring finishes the isolation and cold of winter and prepares the ground for rapid growth and nurture. Sprouting seeds, fresh greens and bright colours, corn yellows, green cabbages, strong colours and fresh individual flavours.

Summer is the season of excess. Foods become over-ripe very quickly. If the sun is too hot then they become engorged and go bad. Summer is the last chance, before the autumn, to lay the ground for new growth but it is also the time of fullness and plenty. Vegetables give way to salads: crisp fresh lettuces, ripe red tomatoes, cucumbers full of liquid flavour, crunchy radish and celery; succulent melon and crisp watermelon, oranges full of flavour and peaches dripping with juice. The colours are fully matured: oranges and pinks, bright greens and pillar box reds. Summer meals tend to consist of rice or pasta with a light sauce. Lots of salads are produced at every meal and fruits are often eaten on their own for dessert with a light cream, fromage frais or even ice cream.

Autumn follows summer all too quickly and autumn uses all the produce left over from summer, decomposing and rotting it to form nourishment for the soil prior to hibernation. Golds, reds and deep oranges are all colours we call autumnal, as in golden apples, deep orange pumpkins and squashes, marrows, potatoes, etc. In autumn we begin the approach to winter by making vegetable soups or lighter soups containing meats and beans – not quite wintery but warming and full of flavour. We tend to stuff things as well – stuffed marrow, stuffed peppers, baked apples and baked potatoes.

Winter is a time of dying off and hibernation. Colours also fade and seasonal foods are warming, in preparation for a long hibernation. We make stews and soups, broths and casseroles, foods that centre on heating us through. We add barley, potatoes and lentils to thicken and give flavour, and we aim to nourish our bodies.

Clearly, eating seasonal foods fulfils all our requirements in terms of nutrition, temperature and taste. It doesn't make sense to chase a piece of salad around a plate in mid-winter and it doesn't make sense to tuck into a hot beef broth on a summer's day.

Working with nature means working naturally, and natural is always best.

STEP 7
Ask for help

Don't let wasteful worry muddy your mind. Remove 'struggle', 'suffering in silence' and 'can't' by simply asking for help.

Any parent will tell you that the constant call of young children is 'Mummy/Daddy, will you help me please?' You stop what you are doing and go over and help. Or you ask them to wait until you have finished what you are up to and then you help them out. You never refuse to give help. They have asked you to help them and so you work out the most convenient time to get together and do just that.

So when did we lose that habit? When did we stop asking for help? Not just help with organising the local jumble sale or help with the school run but help to make a part of our lives more enriching or easier to deal with.

For example, if you have financial concerns and you can't see a way out, getting help may not mean someone giving you money. A friend may offer some fresh ideas to solve the problem, some logistic help to enable you to save or earn more money, or even just a shoulder to cry on. Likewise, needing to find a solution to a gardening problem and knowing someone who has a lovely lawn simply means you give them a call and ask for their help – not free work or favours, but advice.

Having to do something that makes you feel uneasy or apprehensive is always much easier and less daunting if you just express these feelings and ask for help.

The dictionary definition of help is 'assistant and companion, a useful service'. Well, getting a useful assistant to accompany you through something difficult seems a pretty good idea to me.

If you have an idea but don't know how to take it further, find someone whose opinion you value and ask for their help. Asking for help may be difficult but being asked to help someone makes that person feel good. It makes them feel they have a purpose; it calls on their own knowledge or experience; it makes them feel flattered and it means they can help someone out.

Letting something build up inside is exhausting and negative; getting help and moving on is refreshing and uplifting.

Don't be afraid – ask for help and see how good it feels, and then see how good it feels to return the favour when someone asks you for help.

Warning: If you ask for help you may just get it and that could seriously make life easier!

STEP 8
Detox yourself by fasting

Cleanse your insides so that you feel vital, clean, totally detoxed and sparkling, ready to face your world. Fasting will also enable you to clear any over-indulgence in a short space of time, allowing you to get back to full cleanliness and efficiency as soon as possible.

Fasting has been popular for many hundreds of years and claims to be a way of totally cleansing your insides. Fasting means eating nothing and drinking only water. This can be a shock to the system and, unless you really know what you are doing and how you are feeling, it can also be very dangerous. I would advise against anything longer than 48 hours for home fasting.

Fasting allows the body to cleanse waste and empty the system of all residual foods. The clearer the path, the more efficiently the body can absorb and use all the nutrients you take in. Fasting also facilitates the release of hormones that stimulate the immune system.

There are a number of different lengths of fast which can be undertaken but if you wish to complete a fast of two days or more you should always consult your doctor first. Long-term fasting – without correct supervision and instruction – can do more harm than good.

Literally 'starving' your body for more than 24 hours will lead to feelings of weakness, nausea, muscle fatigue, dehydration and dizziness. If you try to operate normally – going to work, looking after the family, and so on – you are likely to suffer major lapses in concentration and extreme fatigue. Any existing health conditions will be exacerbated by lack of nourishment.

There are, however, other forms of fasting that are less severe and, in my view, much more effective. Restricting your diet to certain types of cleansing foods for between 24 and 48 hours can help to detox your system and educate your body into recognising what is good and what is bad.

Once you have fasted and found out how your body reacts to fasting, you may find there are many natural times to fast – when you think that you have eaten too many processed foods or you have had to eat out a lot and don't feel as if you have been very kind to your body. At times like these you can try a mini fast. You can also think about trying a mini-mini fast more regularly, perhaps once a week, on an evening when you are not going out.

If you fast after you have completed a full detox programme it will bring positive results almost immediately. Each time you fast you are just flushing out the small build-up of toxins and waste. Fasting regularly after a complete detox programme will maintain your original detox at its fullest potential.

Fasting must be thought through and preparation is essential if you wish to get the best results. Don't just decide to fast and starve yourself for the next few days – you will find it very unsatisfying.

How to fast

These are the golden rules of fasting:

- Do not fast if you are pregnant or breast-feeding, suffer from any illness, heart condition or diabetes, are taking prescribed drugs, or have doubts about your health.

- Decide when you want to fast and for how long – a mini fast (18 hours) or a mini-mini fast (14 hours).

- *You must start and finish gradually.*

- Leading up to the fast, you should cut out caffeine, processed foods and alcohol – although you have probably already given these up forever!

- The three meals prior to your fast should be light meals consisting of fresh fruit and vegetables, pulses, rice and plenty of fluids.

- Throughout the fast you should:
  - drink plenty of hot water, lemon juice and honey.
  - take vitamin C supplements every four hours and take a timed-release supplement.

– drink at least 3 pints of fluid in the form of water, herbal teas, or apple, grape or lemon juice.

- If hunger becomes unbearable then have to hand some black grapes to nibble on.

Once you have finished your fast, you should again eat only light meals consisting of fresh fruit and vegetables, pulses, rice and plenty of fluids. Then you should slowly reintroduce your normal foods, taking note if anything causes irritation or discomfort. If this occurs then eliminate the irritant foods and detox your diet.

The mini fast (18 hours)

The mini fast can be done once a month and will give your body the 'time out' it needs to cleanse internally. As you can see, the mini fast mainly takes place overnight so you are actually only aware of fasting for around ten hours.

- The mini fast lasts from 6pm in the evening to 3pm the following afternoon.

- Eat only detox foods during the day you start your fast.

- At 6pm eat a light vegetarian meal – ideally from the Detox Your Life programme (see recipes in Chapter 5).

- Eat *nothing* until 3pm the following day but make sure you drink plenty of herbal teas, juices or water during the early evening and following day.

- At 3pm have a light snack of fruit, salad and brown rice.

- At 6pm have another meal of fresh fruit and vegetables.

The mini-mini fast (14 hours)

The mini-mini fast should be done once a week and can probably be done without really noticing you are on a fast! The mini-mini fast takes place from 6pm to 8am the following morning.

As with the mini fast, you are actually asleep for the bulk of the time so it feels like a short four- or five-hour fast. As it is so short you may wonder how it can have any benefits. But even fasting for such a short time gives your body time to process and cleanse.

Getting into the habit of eating your final meal of the day as early as possible will always give your body a better chance to digest your food correctly. Detox or not, the benefits of proper digestion should not be underestimated.

- Eat only detox foods during the day you start your fast.

- At 6pm eat a light vegetarian meal – ideally from the Detox Your Life programme (see recipes in Chapter 5).

- Eat *nothing* until 8am the following day but make sure you drink plenty of herbal teas, juices or water during the early evening.

- At 8am have a light breakfast of hot water and lemon juice, fruit and goat's or sheep's yoghurt and seeds.

- At lunchtime have another meal of fresh fruit and vegetables.

You have now completed a fast with all the benefits and few 'hunger pains'.

NB: This fast is most effective if you have already completed a full dietary detox (either a week-long programme or a full month. See Chapter 4). Perhaps this is the time to try – the details are conveniently covered in the pages ahead.

STEP 9
Water your body

The easiest way to physically and mentally flush away the toxins is to drink plain, simple water. Water your body and watch it grow to full fitness and bountiful energy.

Our bodies are made up of approximately 75 per cent water. Water regulates the function of all our bodily organs and promotes clear skin (the body's largest single organ). During any normal day – not too hot, not too cold, not too active and not too sedentary – we lose about a pint of water through sweating, breathing and evaporation.

In any detox diet you are advised to drink 3 pints or 1.5 litres of water per day.

If possible, this water should *not* be:
- ice cold
- straight from the tap
- from plastic bottles
- filtered by a filter that has not been changed for several months

This water *should* be:
- room temperature
- sourced from a reverse osmosis system that you can attach to your tap at home
- from glass bottles (if bottled)
- drunk regularly on the hour, rather than all at once (in a panic that you have not had enough to drink)

You should increase your water intake gradually. It will take your body a little time to adjust and you will feel that you are spending an inordinate amount of time going to the loo. But once your body has become used to having this fantastic invigorating resource, then it will use it to your best advantage.

If you start feeling thirsty then you are already on your way to the early stages of dehydration – a cause of many small niggles, sicknesses and general tiredness.

Water helps the body to eliminate any waste materials and helps your liver and kidneys to process toxins efficiently. It helps with digestion in the gut and speeds up the detox process all round.

The first response when talking about water intake is usually 'but I drink several cups of tea a day and that has water in it'. The 3 pints or 1.5 litres should come in the form of pure water or herbal teas. Nothing else counts towards your quota – you can have it on top of your daily requirement but certainly not instead of.

One of the first things you notice when drinking the correct amount of water is your increased energy levels.

Then you notice just how clear your skin becomes. There may be a small break-out initially but this is soon cleared up with regular intake.

Then you wonder why you never got this water thing before. With so many benefits, it is just too important to miss out on.

Have a glass and flush away the toxins now.

STEP 10
Clear your mind with meditation

During this Detox Your Life programme you are required to look inwards at yourself and to use your own mind for information that you can work on and work with, to achieve inner peace and calm. Meditation and yoga-style exercise will enhance this process. They can be used throughout the programme and can be continued long after you have completed the programme.

You may think that meditation is a bit 'jingly jangly' and not really for the likes of people with their feet firmly on the ground. Well, not quite so. You would be surprised to find out just how many of your friends, associates and work colleagues have attended or currently attend a class in either meditation or yoga.

Why do so many people pursue this form of relaxation and invigoration? It can aid deep and restful sleep, keep you calm and relaxed even in difficult situations, make you far more creative and inventive, and can also increase your levels of intelligence. With promises like these, you would be silly not to at least give it a serious try.

Meditation can release all tension, relax your system and slow down the thoughts that race through your mind every minute of the day. The meditation process concentrates on the 'now'. Everything that has gone before is irrelevant and everything that is about to happen is ignored. You just stay in the moment, here and now, in a relaxed, calm and meditative state.

The two main types of meditation are Buddhist and Transcendental. Buddhist meditation is similar to positive thinking, and involves thinking good thoughts for the benefit of yourself and others. Transcendental meditation involves sitting in a single position and repeating a saying, phrase or sound until you are entirely absorbed by the meditation process.

Whichever method you choose, meditation is highly appropriate for the Detox Your Life programme because it gives you a total sense of yourself. You can concentrate on clearing your own mind so that you become totally relaxed and at peace with yourself. During meditation, if any everyday concerns enter your mind you simply let them pass and go back to concentrating on the meditation.

Joining a class

Learning to meditate takes a bit of effort – it can be really hard to get into the habit of looking after number one, even if it is only for 20 minutes a day. The best thing to do is to go to a class. These may be held at your local leisure centre or hall. Alternatively, you can call or write to the address on p. 185 and they will inform you where your nearest Transcendental meditation group meets.

Joining a class is beneficial because it immediately puts you together with a group of like-minded people. If you feel part of something it is much easier to get on with it, rather than spending large amounts of time wondering if people think you've gone bananas. Also, on a more serious note, attending a class will help you learn how to use the meditation to get in touch with your own thoughts and how to use that information. Some fairly deep-seated troubles or worries may come out, and a trained teacher can give you support and teach you how best to deal with such issues when you are meditating on your own.

The discipline offered in a class will ensure that the techniques you use are easily understood and keep bringing your mind back to the matter in hand. A class will also help you discover the most appropriate position to meditate in. This is very important, as you can hardly concentrate on your meditation if your legs keep going to sleep or your back is aching. The class will take you through the steps until you feel happy meditating on your own.

Meditating at home

If you wish to meditate at home on your own, here are some important tips:

- Make sure the room is warm and quiet.

- Choose a time when everyone is out and no one is due to call round.

- Put the answerphone on or unplug the phone – if the call is important they will call back. Change your message to let people know you will be available in half an hour.

- Practise using a position that you can stay in for 20 minutes without any discomfort. You may want to lie on your back with your legs and lower back supported by a cushion. Have your arms by your side, with palms facing upwards. Or you may decide to sit cross-legged – this is sometimes helped by placing a cushion under your buttocks so that your pelvis is tilted slightly forwards and your back kept straight. Or you may sit upright with your feet placed sole to sole and your knees simply relaxed and resting on the floor.

- Decide on your mantra or chant. You could start by simply saying your own name in a slow rhythm or just hum to yourself the word 'OM'. Whatever you choose should be low and rhythmic, as the sound is best if it resonates through your muscles as you repeat it.

- Concentrate mainly on your mantra/chant and your breathing. Start with breathing deeply (see 'Correct breathing techniques' below).

- Once you feel relaxed and comfortable, and your breathing is slow and calm, then you should start to chant your mantra slowly and softly until you feel the sound or word resonate through your body.

- Your meditation should only take a short time. If you try to meditate for an hour each day then you will easily find other things that are more pressing. Whereas, if you just meditate for 20 minutes each day, it will be much more practical to schedule. Everyone else can get on with having a cup of tea or emptying the washing machine for those 20 minutes. Then you can emerge, ready to take on the rest of the day, calmer and more relaxed. If at first your family doesn't appreciate you taking 20 minutes for yourself just carry on and they will soon see that you are a much more relaxed person as a result. Before you know it, they will be vacating the house for a full half an hour each day to make sure you get your meditation 'fix'!

Correct breathing techniques

Breathing correctly will help you through every situation you face. Meditation is greatly enhanced if the practitioner is getting the optimum breath for life. Deep breathing can calm and soothe, it can help you gather your thoughts and it can give you balance and concentration.

The following exercise will show you how deep breathing should feel.

- Lie down and place your hands flat on the belly of your stomach with the tips of your fingers just touching.

- Relax your stomach muscles.

- Now inhale through your nose slowly for a count of four. Take in the air until it feels as if the base of your stomach is full of it – this should make your fingertips separate.

- Pause for a count of four, then exhale through your mouth to a count of eight.

Feeling the air 'in your stomach' shows that you have relaxed your diaphragm muscle which means your lungs have fully expanded and you have inhaled to full capacity. This will feel strange at first but will soon become the normal way to breathe and you won't need to think about it any more.

If you feel yourself tensing up or getting nervous then taking ten deep breaths will get you back into a centred position and ready to deal with the situation. Obviously you do not need to lie down to practise deep breathing, but the best way to relax and learn the technique is to try it lying down with no restrictive clothing. Once you know how it feels to take in your full capacity of air, you can breathe correctly all day long.

STEP 11
Detox your space

Enliven your environment, detox unwanted clutter, invigorate yourself, and move forward. Remove everything that gets in the way or is not beautiful or useful.

Space clearing is the art of cleansing and consecrating buildings and homes. This works on two levels: physically and spiritually.

The physical removal of rubbish, dirt and clutter

The most common culprits are old magazines and newspapers, old clothes that you no longer wear, old foods that are past their sell-by date, crockery you don't use, old saucepans that have been replaced by newer, cleaner ones, make-up you never wear, old medicines (that should have been thrown away for safety's sake), old Christmas gift bubble baths that have never been used, the contents of several years of Christmas crackers that you cannot bear to throw away ... Need I say more?

The spiritual removal of stale, stagnant, negative energy or energetic entities (ghosts)

Rooms you don't use, photo albums you have never sorted, thoughts you have never told loved ones, apologies that have gone unheard, confessions not made, secrets not kept ...

Clearing your space

There are many practitioners who would be more than happy to come to your home or office and space clear for you but it might be good to start by seeing how much difference you can make by introducing a few simple techniques yourself.

At its most elementary, space clearing is just like physical spring cleaning. On a deeper level it is about actually cleaning the energy of your home and thus making it fresh and fully active.

- Start by realising that you will not be able to take on the whole house overnight! Clearing should be done thoroughly and systematically – the process should be as ordered and energetic as you wish your home to be once you have completed your clearing.

- Choose a room that you spend most of your time in and then you should feel the benefits of your cleaning immediately. Once you have chosen a room – perhaps your living room – begin. It will be easy to see all the items that can be discarded almost immediately: old postcards, out-of-date magazines, old wrappers, etc. There is nothing scientific in throwing away all the rubbish. The next step is to look at all the items in the room and decide if you really need or want them in there. This is not to say that you should leave your room empty – you may like a lot of furniture. Just make sure that you are only left with useful, practical or beautiful items.

- Once the room is clear of waste, you need to set about physically cleaning it. Vacuum the whole room, move all the furniture and vacuum behind everything and clean away the stale dust that has settled behind the sofa or taken up residence behind the Rembrandt! Polish any surfaces and wipe any windows. Clean the telephone receiver and remove any dead leaves or flowers from house plants.

Check down the side of the chairs for crumbs or coins and 'plump' the cushions. Generally ensure that the room is exactly how you would want it to be if you were arriving home after a long hard day, ready to make you feel welcome and relaxed.

- You can then go on to cleanse the room spiritually, following the instructions below.

   NB: Space clearing will not be understood by everyone, so you should do it when everyone else is out. To encourage the flow and cleansing of energy within your home, you should nurture your home. We talk to our pets, friends and plants. Now it's time to talk to your home.

- Do not attempt space clearing in restrictive clothing. You should wear loose comfortable clothes and relax into your task. You need to be receptive of the 'vibe' you get back from your rooms.

- You can use chimes and bells to clear space; you can use aromatherapy essential oils; and you can use flowers and petals. If the weather is fine you should open the windows and let the air flow. You can use incense or candles to encourage energy to circulate.

- Wander round the room and feel each and every part of it. Identify areas that feel colder and flatter and areas that feel energetic and active. Go around clapping loudly into each and every area to chase out the stagnant energy and move around the active energy – clap low and high.

- Scatter petals or spray essential oils in a water solution lightly around the room. Use a chime to sound in the darkest corners and highest points and move the energy around every nook and cranny. Light candles to draw the air and circulate the atmosphere.

- Before you finish, but after you have worked round every point of the room and energised every angle, you should walk around the perimeter of the room and stroke the energy in an encouraging forward motion – as if encouraging something to pass you by. Once you have done this, the energy should be evenly distributed, cleansed and refreshed.

- Clear away your cleansing equipment – then see how the room feels and how you feel about what you have just achieved.

Search where you will – not a jot of tox will be found, physical, mental or emotional!

STEP 12
Learn to relax and get the best out of stress

Relaxation should be the easiest thing in the world. Just chill out and let it wash over you . . . Once you have detoxed your life, relaxation will be a continual state. That is not to say that you will never do anything or stop responding to outside stimulus; more that everything you do will be done in a way that does not harm your body or put you under any unnecessary stress.

You can be presenting to 500 delegates at a conference or you can stand in a queue at the supermarket with four impatient children and still remain relaxed – if you just use some simple techniques.

The ABC of relaxation

There are many ways to relax and you are bound to know the ones that work best for you but these are usually long-term techniques. Here is an ABC of relaxation that can immediately be applied in moments of shock or anger or just any time when you feel as if things are getting to you. Apply the ABC routine and you can open the doors to total relaxation and detoxification from worry and stress.

Achieve time out

Take five minutes and wander away from the situation. Walk around and tell yourself very simply, in single phrases, what has actually happened. Breaking the situation down into small bite-size pieces makes it easier to digest.

Breathing exercises

Detox the stress by simply breathing correctly. If anything goes wrong or the pressure is getting to you, relax your stomach muscles and breathe deeply into your belly. Breathe in for a count of four, hold the air for a count of four and then release the outward breath for a count of eight. Do this a few times and you will have bought yourself time and space to work out what to do next, or how to react to the situation more beneficially.

Choose to be calm

Make a conscious decision to remain calm and stress-free. As soon as the problem arises or hits you, stop for a second and tell yourself to remain calm, collected and in control. This actually creates a calm state of mind.

Deep relaxation

There are times when we can all benefit from a more thorough detox of stress and strain. The following relaxation exercise will take you away to Planet Detox where everything is perfect and you can return revitalised, calmed and refreshed.

Practice makes perfect but the more you actively practise relaxation techniques, the easier they become; and, as with the following exercise, you will soon be able to take yourself into deep relaxation at any time during the day or night. If you can memorise this sequence or even say it into a tape very slowly and play it to yourself as you are relaxing it may help you carry out the exercise more effectively.

- Find a quiet room. Make sure you are warm and put on some melodic, peaceful music.

- Lie down on the floor or sit comfortably in a chair. Make sure your lower back is supported.

- Close your eyes and start to breathe deeply. Breathe into your belly for a count of four, hold the air for a count of four and then exhale through your mouth for a count of eight.

- After breathing correctly for a couple of minutes you should find that your breathing has slowed down and that it feels very natural.

- Now see in your mind a place that you are very happy in, a place that is relaxing and has powerful feelings of security and enjoyment. It may be a beach you know or a place in the countryside or it may just be your own room at home.

- Take your mind to this place and continue with the exercise whilst you are there.

- Inhale slowly for a count of four and imagine that the air you are breathing is warm and golden and is bathing your body in warm, golden, restful and positive light.

- Now start to consider how your body is feeling. As you inhale, start thinking about your feet and ankles. Are they tense? If so, relax them.

- As you exhale, picture the air you breathe out as old stagnant air and the air you breathe in as new, fresh air.

- Think of your calves and knees and picture the warm air travelling through any tense muscles, bathing them in light. Exhale the stale air.

- Picture your knee joints and your thighs. Breathe deeply and relax. Be aware of your wonderful safe surroundings.

- Feel the fresh air being breathed into the groin area, relaxing the tension and soothing the pelvis. Breathe out the bad air.

- See the golden light swirling around your stomach and abdomen, cleansing and uplifting your centre of emotion and spirit.

- Watch the light thread its way between each and every rib, filling the lungs and chest cavity with warm expanding air.

- Watch every finger fill with golden light and spread through your hands and lower arms.

- Breathe the energy into your shoulders and the base of your neck. Feel your neck relax and melt down into the floor and up into the base of your skull.

- The light may now travel into the root of each and every

hair follicle, making your scalp feel invigorated and tingling.

- Each time you exhale you are breathing out waste. Each time you breathe in you are breathing in new life.

- Now take you mind to the place you have chosen to be and just enjoy all the views, feelings and memories it evokes. Remember how you feel when you are there and how happy and contented you are.

- When you have renewed the life inside your body and you have been in your favourite place for a time, you should move your focus to your new breath, your relaxed body and mind.

- Breathe deeply and inhale all you need.

- Focus on how you feel and how clean your breath is. Focus on your physical body – feel your limbs and feel yourself lying heavily on the floor or bed. Feel your actual surroundings in place of your memory surroundings.

- When you are ready you can start to bring your consciousness back into your own body and into the room you are in.

- Open your eyes slowly. If you are lying on the floor or bed, roll over onto your side and wait a few moments before pushing yourself up to sitting and then standing position.

Feel relaxed, be calmed, centred and grounded – ready to deal with absolutely anything.

STEP 13
Give up smoking

Free your life from the deadly weed and give up smoking. Nicotine is a real physical toxin and right here is where you stop using it.

We all know that smoking is bad for you – it greatly reduces your life expectancy and may even reduce that of those around you. Smoking is one of the greatest self-imposed risks to our lives. STOP SMOKING NOW.

Some more facts, if those are not enough:

- It has been proved that smokers, smoking up to 20 or more cigarettes per day for a two-year period, have considerably more wrinkles than their non-smoking equals.

- Smoking 15 cigarettes a day exposes you to the same amount of radiation as you would get from 150 X-rays a year – the nurses wear lead protection for just one!

- Like caffeine, smoking decreases the body's ability to absorb and use essential vitamins, minerals and amino acids from foods or supplements.

- Of every 1000 young men who smoke cigarettes in England, 250 will be killed prematurely by tobacco (Royal College of Physicians statistics).

- After giving up smoking it takes seven to eight years for the risk of lung cancer to return to the same level as that of non-smokers – the damage to your heart may remain permanently. The risk of heart disease is greater in smokers and ex-smokers than in people who have never smoked in their lives.

- Smoking gives you stale breath and the smoke lingers in your hair, clothes and home.

- Cigarettes are expensive and there are many things we can spend our money on that would help us improve our standard of living rather than reduce the length of our lives.

There are several products on the market, e.g. patches and false cigarettes, and methods such as hypnotism to help you give up. There are also plenty of reasons to do so. Why not detox pollution and toxins from your life, and give up now?

Breathe fresh air into your newly cleansed and truly detoxed life.

STEP 14
Be in the moment

Worrying about the future means you could be worrying about things that may never happen. Detox your life of unnecessary worry by concentrating on what is happening now.

For instance, worrying about trying to pay a bill in August when it is only January gets you nowhere. Planning is useful – worrying is wasted energy.

Worrying about what people may think about something you are going to do next month is wasted energy and can be soul-destroying. Considering all the possible reactions that will affect you and planning how you will deal with them is positive use of energy.

'Being in the moment' is dealing with now. What can you

do about something now? If you cannot do anything now, either plan for when you *can* do something and forget it until then or just stop worrying as there is nothing you can do anyway.

Being in the moment doesn't have to be about problems; it is also about enjoying what you are doing when you are doing it. Here are a few examples:

- Travel to work by train, look at the countryside and feel the movement of the wheels on the tracks – you get to work in the same time but you have a new experience and relax your mind on the way.

- Walk around your garden. Stop thinking about when you will have a chance to mow the lawn and actually notice how fabulous the grass looks now, how it smells now and how the roses smell now, in the cool morning air.

- Eat your lunch and take time to chew your food. Put the sandwich down between each bite and chew each mouthful for at least ten chews. Taste the food. Pick up the sandwich and then take another bite. Think of the food and the nourishment. Don't let your mind wander to the washing up or the report that needs writing or the football match at the weekend. Think of the food whilst you are eating it.

The next time you are doing something that worries you or makes you feel uneasy, take the moment and see how you 'feel' or 'think' in that particular space in time. That way, you may be able to pin down the element that makes you uncomfortable and extract it or change it; and then you can stop worrying.

Being in the moment gives you millions more experiences, feelings and thoughts without having to change a thing. It also gives you a chance to realise how you truly feel and enables you to put into place some plans to stop you having to worry about anything ever again!

How am I feeling now? What can I see now? What am I thinking now? What can I taste now? What can I do now . . . ?

Be in the moment – take time to smell the roses and enrich your life.

STEP 15
Be your own best friend

If you have a friend who is tired, has been through it, been hurt, or is just in need of some support then you think of them and go round to 'help them feel better'. You try to find a way to make sure they 'get up to speed', or 'make a full recovery' or just 'take some time for themselves'.

Well, in order to truly detox your own life, you need to treat yourself as your own best friend. Think about how you feel or about how your life is treating you. If you don't think that you are 'up to speed' or if you have 'been through it' recently then do what you would do for a friend in your situation – but do it for yourself.

Looking back at the cookie jar theory on p. 1, this is a way to start replenishing your own cookie jar.

Take yourself off for a facial, get some aromatherapy, get your bikini line done, take five minutes a day to do some yoga, or buy yourself something.

Anything that you would do for a friend – do for you. In order to start making sure that you are looked after, you should make a list of all the things that you should do or that are overdue but which you will never have the time to do, and then all the things that you would like to try but haven't even dreamt of because of all the other things on the list. Here are some examples:

- Get a haircut

- Get your bikini line done

- Get your roots done

- Get your ingrowing toenail sorted out

- Go to the dentist

- Get your shoes reheeled before they are totally ruined

- Get your eyes checked

- Pick up the dry-cleaning before they sell it on

- Book into a spa for a day

- Book into a spa for a weekend

- Have a bath that lasts longer than half an hour and light some candles, use some oils, etc

- Go shopping for something special – restrict yourself to one item only but make it really special

Make an old friend feel like new – look after you.

STEP 16
Detox your body

Taking care of your body is essential to detoxing your life. If something is not right with our physical being then it impacts on everything we do.

Over the next few days you are going to be setting yourself some great challenges so being able to end the day with a relaxing self-treatment, using yoga, shiatsu, tai chi, aromatherapy, massage or reflexology, is just what you deserve. Take a look at the following and decide to incorporate one treatment a day into the Detox Your Life programme. Then you can promise yourself one treatment a month for the rest of your life – either DIY, or book in for a session with a professional practitioner as a special treat.

Yoga

Yoga is the physical version of meditation. You use your body to effect a change in your whole mind and body. Be warned – yoga is not just a simple form of stretch-and-tone exercise. Some of the advanced moves in yoga look as if they are completely above and beyond the bounds of human flexibility but they really are quite possible if they are taught correctly and you build up to them. Having a relaxed mind will enable your body to 'work out' the moves; attempting them without relaxation is likely to cause injury. After practising yoga for a while you will be able to find emotional, physical and mental calm.

Yoga will tone your external body but it will also tone your internal systems (respiratory, circulatory, lymph, etc). It will also work your internal organs, as some of the positions will exert pressure on or release pressure from them and their surrounding areas. It will stretch your muscles, keep your joints supple and your spine healthy, supportive and strong. Each position has its own purpose. A yoga sequence or session will work all aspects of the body and free everything up so that you achieve mental and physical clarity. Breathing into moves and holding them requires concentration and balance. There is nothing quick or sharp about yoga.

As with meditation, you should always start by attending a class or having lessons with a qualified, experienced yoga teacher.

Tai chi

Tai chi dates back to ancient China – as far back as 3000 BC. Only now, nearly 5000 years later, have we Westerners decided that there may be something in it! Tai chi literally means 'big energy'. It involves becoming aware of our own personal energy and the energy surrounding us, and harmonising them to produce more energy.

Everything has energy – we just need to do some elementary work to start to recognise how it manifests itself and how we can harness it for ourselves. Tai chi is also exercise and, through the energy generated by some graceful balletic movements, we begin to feel the flow of energy – both personal and surrounding.

As with all Oriental treatments, there are a few basics to get to grips with, and sequences to follow to get your energy to flow and ebb, and then you can practise tai chi safely almost anywhere you wish.

In China, many people go out to an open space – parks, gardens, poolsides – and practise there. The energy or 'chi' actually changes at around 3 or 4am every morning, and devout practitioners will tell you that dawn exercise is one of the most amazing ways to experience tai chi. However, it is perhaps a little more practical to begin your foray into tai chi in a class, or your own home or gym, in order to feel comfortable before you 'go public'.

Shiatsu

Shiatsu is another Oriental art, working with the body to increase energy flow and health.

The Chinese use acupuncture and acupressure; the Japanese employ shiatsu (which involves exerting firm pressure on different points of the body that relate to different energy paths or specific organs – in a very similar way to the meridians used in acupuncture and reflexology).

Pressure physically applied to points of the body, using elbows, knees, fingers and many other parts of the body, will invigorate the client and clear any blockages in energy that are causing an imbalance, thus resulting in fitness and balanced flow.

Aromatherapy

If you are going to take on the task of detoxing your mind, then it is only right that you should use all the support and help you can get.

Aromatherapy (using essential oils) is one of the ways that you can have this support with you at all times.

NB: Essential oils should never be used if you believe you are pregnant or if you are trying to become pregnant, unless otherwise prescribed by a trained aromatherapist. Essential oils should never be taken internally. Aromatherapy oils are not to be taken lightly, as they can be dangerous if used incorrectly or in the wrong amounts. They are not just nice-smelling oils (as some people believe) but strong, effective drugs that can have both subtle and huge effects on the body, mind and emotions. Use these oils with caution, and under instruction from a qualified aromatherapist or following the advice in a book or leaflet. You should never just choose an oil because it has a pleasant aroma; it may have harmful or dangerous side effects or contraindications.

The market has become much more aware of essential oils over the last few years and now many, many products are available that make using essential oils much safer and more practical. There are ready-made blends of essential oils, ready-made blends of bathing/massage oils and even ready-made sprays of essential oils and carrier oils to keep with you and just use as required. The element of doubt when using pure essential oils can be eliminated when using these blends but you may still wish to try using a small number of essential oils to create your own blends. If you do so, *always* follow the instructions.

During the Detox Your Life programme you will be undertaking some interesting and unusual tasks and the support of essential oils will enhance the programme and speed up the detox process. There are many ways to use essential oils at home and you should try all of them over the next few days so you can work out which one best suits you and your lifestyle.

After you have completed the programme you are likely to have found some oils that you will keep with you always and that can help you through any situation or give you an instant boost.

Aromatherapy/essential oils and massage

When used at home without the instruction of a trained therapist, essential oils should never be applied directly to the skin without first being diluted. Essential oils are highly concentrated and can cause irritation or burning when applied undiluted or undispersed. (More than a ton of petals can be required to provide just 2ml of essential oil.)

Carrier oils or base oils can be used as a blend. Many of these are simply natural vegetable or seed oils that we use every day in our kitchens. This may seem a bit crude but the oils are totally natural and therefore can be absorbed by the skin and act as a moisturiser. Olive oil, sunflower oil, safflower oil, grapeseed oil, nut oil and sesame oil are all natural, readily available oils that can be used. Macadamia nut oil, sweet almond oil, jojoba oil or avocado oil are slightly more exotic and can be found in natural health stores or some more enlightened chemists. These are just as good if not better but are less readily available. All carrier or base oils will dilute the stronger, more potent essential oil and this will decrease the chance of skin irritation.

The ratio of any home-made blend of massage oils should be no more than eight drops of essential oil to every 20ml of carrier or base oil. You should only blend sufficient oils for immediate use. Essential oils are a natural preservative but if stored incorrectly the blend can become stale or rancid.

Find a plastic bottle or bowl and pour in 20ml of base oil. Add your desired essential oil, drop by drop to your base oil and stop when the blend has a sufficiently strong fragrance for your taste. Some oils are stronger than others and you may only use two or three drops in total. But never use more than eight drops per 20ml – it is always better to have less essential oil than more, as using too much can sometimes cause headaches.

Use the blend as you would normally use oil in a self-massage.

If you have a professional aromatherapy massage you will be asked to lie on a massage couch, either naked or in your underwear, covered in towels or blankets to keep warm. The room should be warm and the practitioner should have a calm, relaxing approach. The treatment will usually last about an hour. You may feel drowsy after the session but a glass of water will soon remedy this.

When the massage is complete, try to keep the oil on your skin for a minimum of an hour as this will allow the essential oil to continue being absorbed. If you need to dress after a massage then wipe off any excess oil before dressing as the oil may colour or stain your clothing.

Aromatherapy/essential oils and bathing

As with massage, essential oils should never be used without being first diluted in base or carrier oils (see above), or dispersed in a dispersant.

Dispersants can be found in the house and the two most readily available ones are milk or high-volume alcohol (vodka is best as it has no fragrance and no sugar residue). These products will break down the essential oil into much smaller droplets which means the oil is more evenly spread in the water and is less likely to cause irritation to the skin.

Diluting your essential oil with a base or carrier oil will make your bath more oily. This is great if you can massage the residue of oil into your skin after the bath but if you need to dress immediately afterwards then a dispersant is more practical. It will allow the oil to be immediately absorbed into the skin without leaving a greasy residue.

When bathing in oils you should not attempt to use soap

or bubble bath for washing, as this will destroy the effect of the natural oil. Choose a time when you do not need to wash (i.e. just before bed or after you have taken a quick shower). Run a bath that is hot enough to stay warm for 15–20 minutes but not so hot that it is uncomfortable to sit in.

Choose either to dilute or disperse your essential oil. Whatever you choose – dispersant or carrier oil – you need only fill a tablespoon with your chosen fluid. You will only need to add between two and four drops of essential oil to this.

When the bath is full, sprinkle the tablespoon of blended oil over the water.

Close all the windows so that none of the steam escapes. You might also want to light some candles for a really relaxing, sensuous experience. Slowly get into the bath and, once in, concentrate on breathing slowly and deeply, inhaling all the vapour from the oil. Allow your skin to soak and absorb all the oils. You should be able to totally relax and unwind, and to detox your mind.

Once you have finished the bath, get out slowly. If you have used a carrier oil, try to collect all the oil from the surface of the water onto your skin. Pat yourself dry, allowing as much of the oil as possible to stay on your flesh, acting as a natural moisturiser. Any residual oil will continue to be absorbed.

Ideally, you can now relax or go straight to bed!

Aromatherapy/essential oils and inhalations

Using essential oils for inhalations is an excellent way to benefit from essential oils immediately without removing any clothing.

When you breathe in the vapour from the oils they enter

the olfactory system instantly so attention should be paid to amounts used. As with many natural therapies, the correct dose will solve a problem but using too much will often exacerbate the problem.

Very much like any 'grandmother's remedy', you need to boil some water and pour it into a large bowl. Add two or three drops of your chosen oil (no dispersants or carriers are required as the oil does not come into direct contact with the skin). Then lower your head, covered with a towel or sheet, over the bowl. Inhale slowly through your nose and out through your mouth, lowering your face closer to the water as you become used to the vapour. Inhaling is an excellent method for colds and coughs as the effects are immediate. Inhale for about five minutes or until you have had enough, then uncover your head and breathe the cool air.

You can also inhale oils by placing two or three drops on an old handkerchief (the oils may stain). Holding the cloth near your nose or mouth, you can inhale in the same way. Do not hold the cloth directly on your skin, as the oils may irritate.

Aromatherapy/essential oils and compresses

There are some times when nothing more than a hot water bottle is required to relieve discomfort or pain or to simply give warmth and comfort. Using a compress is aromatherapy's answer to this.

You need to fill a large bowl with hand-hot water, add a couple of drops of your chosen essential oil to the water and soak a large piece of cotton cloth for a couple of minutes. Wring out the cloth and fold it into a compress large enough to cover the area of discomfort. Add two further drops of your oil directly onto the compress (it will spread and dilute into the soaked cotton) and then hold the compress onto the area of pain. You can use the compress until it cools down and if you wish you can repeat the process.

The compress is an ideal treatment for period pains, fever and headaches, though you can of course use the compress for any condition or any reason. A lavender and ylang ylang compress (both oils for relaxation and rejuvenation), held against the forehead, is particularly soothing.

Aromatherapy/essential oils and burners

Oil burners are an excellent way of getting essential oils into the atmosphere so that you can benefit from their therapeutic qualities whilst you go about your everyday business.

NB: oils should not be used when there are children under five in the room or house.

When choosing your burner you need to get one with a bowl that is big enough to contain 120ml of water. If the bowl holds much more than this then it will take too long to heat the water; and if the bowl is much smaller then it will have burnt dry, giving a rancid smell, before the candle has gone out. You need to fill the burner with water, light the candle below and then drop four or five drops of your chosen oil onto the surface of the water. You are unlikely to use too much oil in a burner, as the vapour is distributed throughout the building. But if you start to develop a mild headache simply add more water or blow out the candle.

Alternatively, you could use dry burners – the terracotta rings that go on light bulbs or the electrically heated porcelain plates. When a few drops of your chosen oil are placed on the heated surface, the heat causes them to evaporate, releasing the fragrance. They can be controlled by turning off the power or removing the terracotta burner.

Aromatherapy/essential oils and ready-made blends

Ready-made blends are the complementary therapy answer to using essential oils quickly, relatively inexpensively and safely.

If people decide to use essential oils at home after reading a short book about them, they run the risk of causing quite a lot of damage. It is human nature to add our own personal interpretation to anything but when using essential oils any creativity can be dangerous. When baking a cake, for example, you might decide to add more orange zest than the recipe suggested to boost the flavour and colour. This would probably make your cake even more delicious. However, if you were to apply the same principle in creating an essential oil blend – perhaps adding more basil because you like the smell – then the blend would take on a completely different quality and might well aggravate the problem rather than solve it.

Ready-made blends are therefore an excellent way to try aromatherapy without any risk of getting it wrong. However, there are many different aromatherapy products available, of varying degrees of potency.

If you look at the products available in the shops you can always use colour to help make your decision as to how natural they are, and how much of the essential oil they actually contain. For example, if you pick a relaxing blend for massage containing lavender and other relaxing oils then the blend should be of neutral colouring, not bright blue or dark green. If you want a bath oil to invigorate then a bright pink or orange one is only likely to perk you up if you look at it rather than bathe in it! This is not to say that there is no place for these products. It is great that people are being made more aware of the properties of aromatherapy oils; they are wonderful gifts, and if they make you take a bath or have a massage then that has many benefits. However if you wish to use essential oils for their specific, therapeutic qualities then you really need to use the pure essential oil in a carrier or base oil.

Around 99 per cent of essential oils are a clear, light yellow colour; some go as far as deep orange (e.g. neroli and mandarin); and some are very light, almost transparent (e.g. lavender). Very few, and certainly very uncommon oils, are what we would call coloured (blue chamomile is an incredibly dark blue, an almost inky colour). So it is fair to say that most of the oils you would come across for day-to-day use are light yellow. Carrier or base oils are the same, they are all varying degrees of yellow to mid-brown. Grapeseed is slightly greener and nut oils are very dark brown but all are natural/neutral.

The essential oils you need for the Detox Your Life programme are:

Rose

Rose is one of the most expensive oils but also one of the most amazing and magical. Rose has anti-inflammatory properties and is great for 'feminine' conditions, such as PMS, anorexia, and stomach cramps. This is a real treat but incredibly beneficial.

Rosemary

Rosemary is a great stabiliser. It keeps your mind clear and soothes away tension headaches and stress – just the right oil for changing your life.

Geranium

Geranium balances. If you are hyper it calms you down and if you are down it perks you up. Ideal for hormone imbalance, depression and general mood swings.

Juniper

Juniper is a special detox oil, as it helps the body to cleanse itself. It is a diuretic and has amazing antiseptic properties.

Eucalyptus

Eucalyptus will also kill all known germs dead, so when you are feeling at a low ebb, kick in with this oil and feel the benefit. It will also stimulate and invigorate, and banish the nasty itching caused by insect bites and stings.

Chamomile

Chamomile tea is famous for relaxing the mind and body; chamomile essential oil does exactly the same. It has a calming effect, physically and mentally, and will help you sleep through the night and face the next day of the Detox Your Life programme with renewed vigour.

Reflexology

Reflexology is based on the principle of reflex points or zones on the feet relating to points, organs and systems within the body. By working with these zones or points, the practitioner can treat areas of illness, imbalance or weakness.

Reflexology has been recorded as far back as ancient Egyptian times and Eunice Ingham documented the practice in the early 1900s.

During a reflexology treatment the client is required to sit or lie on a treatment couch and the practitioner will follow a sequence around each foot that covers every reflex point or zone. The practitioner will require feedback from the client concerning areas of discomfort or pain during the treatment; the practitioner can then 'work' the relevant area to improve the condition. Reflexology practitioners tend to use powders to make the treatment go smoothly, such as calendula or talcum. Reflexology is an excellent diagnostic tool, as it can show any problems, even at the early stages, within the body. The practitioner can then work on them before any further, more serious conditions develop.

During the Detox Your Life programme your internal systems and organs will probably be working harder or differently from the way they normally do. Reflexology can help by 'balancing' organs like the kidneys and liver, and enabling the intestines to carry out their cleansing functions without causing any unnecessary pressure or imbalance. Reflexology can also tell you what your body requires or simply what it is going through. If you have reflexology treatments whilst you are detoxing you will find that common 'tender points' are those of the bladder, kidneys and digestive systems, all of which are working hard. The practitioner will work on these specific points to bring them to optimum condition for continued cleansing.

Reflexology treatments will also show up any potential imbalance so that the practitioner can work at a preventative level. If you are super-healthy, or your detox has made your body totally balanced, then reflexology treatments are still useful as a maintenance precaution and for relaxation.

There are also some elementary reflex points that you can work on yourself every day to achieve calm and full healthy balance:

- The first one is often called The Great Eliminator because it is a trigger point that will help to expel stress and tension. The Great Eliminator is located in the fleshy part of your hand between thumb and forefinger. Using the thumb and forefinger of your left hand, gently squeeze this fleshy area on your right hand. You should apply pressure slowly, as it may well be tender especially if you have a headache or are tense. Hold the pressure and release slowly, then repeat until you feel the tension or the headache subside. When you feel ready, swap hands and release tension on the other hand.

- The centre point of the palm of your hand relates to the centre point of your solar plexus (chest area) and the centre point on your foot. Obviously the easiest point to reach is your hand so you can work this area without anyone ever knowing. Place your left thumb in the centre of your right palm, supporting the weight of the right hand with the fingers of the left. Slowly move the thumb upwards towards the fingers and stop when you meet the underside of the knuckles (just off-centre from the palm towards the fingers). Again apply pressure slowly and hold it until the pressure subsides. Repeat for the other hand and feel the tension melt away.

- You can also apply pressure to the zone points on the face by placing both thumbs just inside the eye sockets, up against the brow bone. Place your elbows on your desk or a table and then lower the weight of your head onto your thumbs. Again, this may feel tender especially if you are trying to eliminate a headache. Hold the pressure and then release.

Massage

Massage is natural and free of charge, and you can do it to yourself any time you want to. The 'laying-on of hands' has been used for hundreds of years, and the formal 'massage' treatment as we know it has become increasingly popular in recent years, as people have taken more responsibility for their own health and fitness.

On a basic level, massage increases circulation, warms the flesh, lowers blood pressure and helps us produce endorphins – the body's natural 'feel-good' hormones.

Touch, through massage, can make you feel safe, cared for, healthy and relaxed. As the massage strokes work over your body, you begin to feel your muscle fibres relax and the tension disappears. The adrenaline stored in the muscles at the shoulder and in the back of the legs is passed into the body's natural waste disposal system. All the toxic build-up begins to break down into a size that the body can deal with efficiently and effectively.

Massage can not only be relaxing and rejuvenating but also wonderfully healing. Feeling every aspect of your body and connecting them back with each other during the massage means that you emerge whole and centred once again and ready to face the world.

Follow the self-massage techniques described in Step 18 (p. 104) and convert yourself to a thoroughly massaged and relaxed being . . .

**Whatever form of treatment you choose,
feel the tox melt away and your body thank
you for the treat.**

STEP 17
Wash away the toxins

Spas are appearing all over the UK and Europe, reflecting the increasing popularity of hydrotherapy, another form of therapy dating back to ancient times. Hydrotherapy enables you to wash away the toxins and splash your way to a cleaner, healthier you.

Flotation tanks

Flotation tanks are great for unwinding and shutting out the outside world. You get into a tank of salinated water which is only a few inches deep, but because of the salt content you float on the surface. The room or tank is dark, and once the music starts to pipe through you really do lose your sense of anything except the sensation of floating – hence the name.

The flotation tank instils a feeling of peace, calm and rest and even after a 20-minute session you feel as if your troubles have just floated away.

Watsu

Watsu treatments are relatively new and consist of a shiatsu-like massage sequence whilst you are suspended in water. Throughout the treatment you are totally supported by the practitioner and the ballet-like stretches you perform again make you feel as if you are floating or flying. The watsu treatment takes place in a heated swimming pool, so when you fully relax into the treatment, the caressing from the practitioner and the heat from the pool really make you feel that you are floating on air – a very womb-like experience.

Aqua aerobics

Aqua aerobics is the same as normal aerobics but you take the class in the water. This enables more extreme movements without causing any pressure on joints, as the water fully supports the body. The exercise element is increased, as running in the pool means that you are pushing against several gallons of water. This is a very safe way to build muscle tone and increase aerobic capacity and strength.

Bathing and soaking

Bathing is a greatly underestimated part of hydrotherapy, and washing the body is a very sensual and essential part of body care. Many religions use washing and cleansing as a ritual before any worship and in some cultures the greatest compliment you can pay someone is to wash their feet for them. So next time you run a bath, don't just go for a quick scrub down, allow your skin to soak and soften and then apply exfoliation scrubs (see p. 108) and wonderful moisturisers (see p. 112).

Sea water therapy

Thalassotherapy (the Greek word *thalassa* meaning 'sea') uses sea water and salinated water in many different ways. It has been around for thousands of years, but is now becoming increasingly popular. Sea water contains many minerals, and wraps and potions derived from it are of great benefit in body care and cleansing. The sea water contains elements very similar to our own blood plasma and that is why the body feels so at home in marine environments. The body absorbs these elements during thalassotherapy treatment and uses their health-giving and restorative properties.

Turkish baths

Turkish baths, which consist of steaming, sauna and body rub-downs, followed by rigorous massage and application of oils, thoroughly cleanse the skin and promote a sense of calm and relaxation.

Blitz showers

Blitz showers use strong jets of hot and cold water to increase circulation and massage the flesh. The practitioner will place you at the end of a tiled corridor and ask you to face forwards, side on and backwards as she applies jets of water of differing strengths to your torso. This treatment can be slightly painful as you adjust to the strength of the jet and the heat/cold of the water but by the end you will feel invigorated and purged of both surface and deep toxins.

Colonic irrigation

Colonic irrigation has been around since 1500 BC, but most people think of it as a relatively new and experimental therapy.

Essentially, it is an internal bath that helps to cleanse the colon of accumulated poisons, gases, faecal matter and mucous deposits. The practitioner will gently pump filtered water into the rectum and this will start to soften and flush away any build-up of toxins and waste.

Colonic irrigation is extremely effective during the Detox

Your Life programme. During the programme you eliminate any sources of toxins from your diet. However, there will still be a build-up of toxins within the body from prior to the programme. The foodstuffs you are eating, such as brown rice, nuts and pulses, all help to break this down, but colonic irrigation will speed up the process and will actively flush out any matter.

The colonics practitioner will ask you to lie on a couch or plinth, with your lower body covered with a towel or sheet. Filtered water at a carefully regulated temperature is introduced under gentle gravitational pressure through the rectum and into the colon. The practitioner will use massage to help the water soften and cleanse the colon of faecal matter that is flushed away with the waste water. The colon is worked on in stages; each time, the water is pumped in and flushed out until the whole area is complete. The treatment lasts less than an hour and the modesty of the client is observed throughout. It is then usual for the practitioner to recommend how many further treatments are required and also which supplements you need to take to replace natural bowel fibre and flora.

The after-effects of colonic irrigation are similar to those of the entire detox programme: a feeling of well-being, lightness, mental clarity, increased energy, loss of bloated feeling, relief from constipation, and clearer, glowing skin.

If you have ever thought about having this treatment then this is the time to try! It's painless, it's different, it makes you feel great and it is detoxifying.

Splash your way to renewed vigour and wash away any hint of worry – cleanse and revitalise!

STEP 18
Slough, scrub and purge

The Detox Your Life programme is a thorough way to keep your body in the best possible condition from both the outside and the inside. To enhance the vitality of your body and mind, you should follow this body care routine:

Cold shower every morning
Wakes you up, stimulates your circulation and leaves you with a warm glow all day long.

Dry skin brush every morning
Detoxes the dead skin cells and lets your body take a deep uninhibited breath.

Exfoliate every three days
Cleanses the toxins from your skin and shows how banishing the bacteria leads to a beautiful fresh face.

Have an Epsom salts bath every five days
Epsom salts (or magnesium) drain the toxins away as you lounge in a deep relaxing bath.

Moisturise fully
Drinking hydrates the inside and moisturisation helps from the outside.

Self-massage every morning and evening
Tones the skin, tones the muscles, smooths the flesh and banishes cellulite!

See the following pages for details of how to give your body all these wonderful treats.

Cold shower

An invigorating swim in a cool pool, sea or lake every morning would be an ideal scenario. But if you needed to include a long cool swim every day, alongside all your other new activities, you would soon find yourself spending more time detoxing and less time living your life! Here's an alternative that takes two minutes and gives you all the benefits of the swim without having to leave your own home: a cold shower!

This may sound mad but if you have ever taken a shower or bath somewhere where there was no hot water you may remember that it was a most invigorating experience that actually left you feeling considerably warmer than a normal hot shower. Indeed, it is more effective in hot weather to take a lukewarm shower (rather than a cold one) as a cold shower will increase your circulation and warm you up, not cool you down.

When bathing or showering in the mornings, simply turn the shower to cold just before you are ready to finish and let the icy cold water run over your entire body for one minute. Alternatively, when you have finished your bath, you can turn on the cold tap as the bath water is draining away, cup your hands under the water and splash it all over your body.

If you happen to live by the sea then any chance you get you should take off your shoes and paddle for two minutes tops – we don't want any reports of frostbite!

Dry skin brushing

This once unheard of process now leaps out of every health magazine article – and quite right too! Sloughing away dead skin cells helps your skin 'breathe' efficiently. It also clears the pores, and improves the appearance of the skin (dead skin is dull and does not reflect light well, whereas healthy skin glows in normal light conditions).

Brushing improves blood and lymph circulation. The action of brushing stimulates muscle contraction to help the lymph and blood flow.

The improved lymph flow makes the excretion of waste materials in the cells and interstitial fluid more efficient. Clearing this area also encourages cell production and renewal.

Increasing the flow of interstitial fluid in turn causes excess fluids to drain and clear from the troublesome hip and thigh areas. Pooling, water retention or oedema can thus be prevented with more efficient fluid and lymph flow.

Brushing also stimulates the production of sebum which helps to improve the texture and tone of the skin.

Now that you have plenty of excellent reasons to dry skin brush, you need to know how to do it effectively:

• Find a natural bristle brush, loofah, a dry flannel or mitt. The bristles or flannel should be firm but not hard. You will be brushing your skin quite vigorously all over your body – and the skin on your stomach is softer than the skin on your shins or forearms. Do not wet or moisturise the skin, as this may cause dragging.

• Having undressed to your underwear or preferably with no clothes on at all, stand or sit in a position that enables access to all parts of your body. Sitting on the edge of the bath with one foot up on the toilet seat or sitting on the edge of the bed with your feet on pillows is quite good.

- Start at the feet and systematically work your way up towards the top of your body. All strokes should be towards the heart. The heart easily pumps the blood down throughout the body but both blood and lymph need extra help to work against gravity to return through the system. (Brushing away from the heart may cause faintness or disrupt the normal flow.) Each stroke should be long and firm. Place the brush/mitt on your ankle and firmly brush up to your knee. Repeat until you have covered the entire calf and shin several times. When you have completed the lower leg, move up to the knee. The next strokes should run from the knee to the top of the thigh and over the buttocks.

- Then brush both arms from the wrist to the shoulder. The neck and shoulder area should be treated more gently, as the flesh here is very delicate. Work from the top of the arm, up and over the shoulder and gently up the neck to the base of the skull.

- When brushing the stomach, use gentle circular strokes in a clockwise direction. This will follow the flow in your intestines and will not disrupt any bowel functions.

- You must only brush the face with a soft facial brush or flannel as the skin on the face is very delicate and can be damaged if the brush is too hard.

The whole process should only take three or four minutes and you should feel quite invigorated when you have finished. Your skin will tingle and you should feel warm, as you will have stimulated and increased your circulation. You will soon notice quite a difference in your skin. It should feel smoother with a softer texture, and the dry patches will all have disappeared. Just spend a little time each day and you will be pleasantly surprised.

Exfoliation

Dry skin brushing is quick and convenient if you are including it in your morning routine before you have to take the children to nursery or dash off to work (or if you simply want a great wake-up energy booster). Exfoliation has all the same benefits but it can be included as part of the more relaxing, more tranquil – or even indulgent – times in your detox programme. Exfoliation needs water and some form of home-made or cosmetic exfoliant. Exfoliation is generally gentler on the skin and it can therefore be used on the face and any delicate areas that might find dry brushing a little too harsh. Exfoliating products are widely available in all price ranges and are usually combined with wonderful-smelling creams or gels. However, if you do not wish to buy an exfoliating scrub then you can easily make your own.

Home-made exfoliating mix (enough for one bath/scrub)

1 tablespoon salt flakes
(You can use normal salt if your skin is delicate or if you want a less rigorous product)
2 tablespoons vegetable or seed oil (e.g. olive, sunflower, sesame, etc)
1 tablespoon honey

Place all the ingredients in a plastic bowl and mix together until you have a runny paste. Dip the ends of your fingers into the pot and scoop about a teaspoon of the mix out each time. Rub this all over the body and apply more when required. (The salt is the exfoliant and the oil and honey will help to moisturise the flesh.)

Alternatively, you can turn your favourite body oil into an exfoliant by simply adding the salt to a small amount of your chosen product and then use as described below.

You can exfoliate in the bath or shower but unless you have a palatial shower then you may find that the cream has been washed off before you get the chance to benefit from the exfoliating properties. Ideally you should exfoliate during a nice relaxing bath. Here's how:

• Run a bath and put a few drops of your favourite bath oil or foam into the water. Get in and relax! Allow at least ten minutes before you start to exfoliate, as this will give you time to relax and give your skin time to soften with the water/oils etc.

There are now two options:
    You can exfoliate out of the bath or in the bath.

• To follow the first option, get out of the bath, making sure the bathroom is still nice and warm. Gently rub your exfoliating cream or home-made exfoliant in firm, large and small circles all over your body. Pay special attention to any areas of hard skin – heels, knees, elbows, etc – and rub as hard as you find comfortable. The whole process should take about three or four minutes. When you have completed the 'rub', get back into the bath and carry on the circular rubbing until all the cream has been washed off into the bath water. Get out of the bath and rub yourself dry with a towel (one that has *not* been rinsed in fabric conditioner as this will increase its absorbency and will carry on the exfoliating process as you are drying yourself). Once dry, apply a good moisturiser or body oil all over the body and stay warm. Going to bed with a good book or having an early night is simply your best bet here!

- To follow the second option, stay in the bath and lift each limb above the surface of the water. Exfoliate as described before, in firm, large and small circles. As you finish each limb, lower it back into the water and continue to work the flesh until all the cream has been washed away. The only area that may get neglected using this method is that of the buttocks but you can do this area by kneeling up in the bath. Towel dry as before and then moisturise and keep warm.

Epsom salts baths

Magnesium is essential for nearly all our bodies' cellular activity, and bathing in Epsom salts allows the skin to absorb magnesium. The magnesium will also absorb or 'draw' toxins from the body, so it is likely that you will glow with perspiration for a while after your bath. This will not be quite like a sweat – unless you wrap up really warm! It is more likely to feel as if you are in a very humid room. It is very important to keep warm, not only to increase the effect of the magnesium but also to avoid catching a chill. Epsom salts baths improve circulation and speed up the elimination of toxins.

An Epsom salts bath can also be extremely relaxing and warming, helping to soothe aching joints and muscles. Taken before bed, this will almost certainly guarantee the deepest night's sleep.

To make the ideal Epsom salts bath:

- Buy your Epsom salts from a chemist or health food shop.

- Run a deep bath that is warm enough to sit in comfortably for 10 to 15 minutes without going cold. Pour about 2lb (1kg) of Epsom salts (it is a lot but you need this much to get the best effect) into your bath and stir until it has all dissolved. Get into the bath and have ready a loofah glove or massage mitt.

- Sit in the bath for at least five minutes before you start to massage your body. Start massaging with slow gentle strokes, and as you get more used to this make the strokes more rigorous. It is likely that you will feel very warm quite quickly as the magnesium has a warming effect. If this happens, slow down your massage and just let the Epsom salts work on you as you relax.

- When you get out of the bath then you should pat yourself dry and wrap up warm for the next hour or so. Ideally, the bath should be taken in the evening just before you are about to go to bed, which will keep you warm for many hours. Alternatively, you can take the bath during the day and wrap up in a quilt or blanket and sit and watch an old movie!

Don't be surprised if you feel quite tired after an Epsom salts bath, as it will be having a major effect on your internal systems – all for the good.

For best results, you should take an Epsom salts bath every three days during the Detox Your Life programme, but don't take one if you suffer from any skin condition or have any cuts or grazes.

Moisturising

During the programme you will be doing many new and different things to your body, most of which will require an increased level of activity either internally or externally. During all these processes – exercise, sweating, cell regeneration, elimination of toxins and cleansing – your body will be using up fluids. It is imperative to replace these fluids so that your body can maintain optimum levels of detoxing.

We already know that we need to drink at least 3 pints (1.5 litres) of water per day to keep our fluid levels steady. But we also need to make sure that all other areas of moisture are maintained.

Creams and gels are not the only way to preserve the skin's natural moisture levels – oils are just as effective, if not better.

Each time you bathe, wash, receive a treatment or carry out any of the detox body care treatments, you should remember to moisturise your skin afterwards.

A daily skin care routine is essential if you wish your skin to stay in optimum condition. It is better to do a little and do it often (e.g. simply wash with water and follow with a moisturiser every day) than to do a lot infrequently (e.g. cleanse, tone, scrub, face mask, exfoliate once a month).

Keeping your skin, body and facial moisture levels up is important for the detox process. It will also give your skin a warm glow, allow it to shed old dead cells more effectively, and prevent it from looking dry and dull.

Self-massage

I could go on for days about how good massage is for everything! But I will stick to the specific ways in which massage can enhance the detox process.

It would be wonderful if we could all have massage treatments every day of our lives but it takes time and money and a lot of practitioners! Self-massage avoids all these problems. It is cheap, completely portable and can be done any time and anywhere. So why is massage so good for detox? It:

- Warms and relaxes the muscles

- Relieves tension

- Aids stress reduction

- Stimulates blood circulation

- Increases lymph flow

- Improves the immune system

- Helps the body eliminate excess fluids and waste products

- Improves the flow of interstitial fluid, improving the appearance of the skin, especially in areas prone to cellulite

- Lowers blood pressure

- Tones muscles and skin

- Provides a passive workout for the whole body

Most normal massage strokes can be converted to be used for self-massage. As long as you observe the general rules of massage, even 'made up' strokes will be perfectly acceptable and effective.

1. As with dry skin brushing (see pp. 105–108) *all massage strokes should be towards the heart* (venous return). The blood should be pushed around the system in conjunction with the circulation and not against it.

2. *Always use either the flat hand* (fingers together, palms down) *or the ends of the fingers* (bunched together, no fingernails!).

3. *All massage strokes should start lightly and slowly build to a firmer, more rapid pace.*

4. *The flesh should be warm and relaxed* before any deeper strokes can be used. Working deeply on cold, tense flesh will feel unpleasant and can cause bruising.

5. *Massage should never be painful or sore* but massage that is too light is little better than a comforting stroke.

6. *You should be relaxed* when carrying out self-massage, as you need to work in some awkward positions and do not want to cause any twists or injuries.

You should massage yourself every day during the detox programme. As this can become time-consuming, the full massage has been broken down into sequences. Try to do at least two of the sequences each day and this will ensure that over a week you will get a full body treatment. Remember, take it slowly at first. As your knowledge and confidence build, you will be able to make adjustments as necessary.

Make sure the room you are in is warm and quiet – perhaps with some relaxing, calming music playing. If the room is cold you will not be totally relaxed and this is not going to result in the best massage.

You should use a massage oil, favourite cream or body lotion and apply just enough to allow your hands to work over the flesh firmly. If you use too much you will just slip over the skin and if you use too little you may pull or burn the skin. If you apply too much just wipe the excess onto another part of the body where you can use it later.

Face and neck sequence

Place the pads of your fingers together and press them onto your face quite firmly.

Working together, circle both hands upwards, outwards and down, all over the surface of your face – remember to work your cheeks, forehead, nose, lips, etc.

Relax your jawbone and let your mouth relax.

Continue the strokes down your neck and over the front of your chest in small and large circles.

Shoulder and arm sequence

Place a flat hand onto your lower arm. Keeping as much of your hand as possible on the arm, work in long, smooth, firm strokes from the base of the arm, up and over the shoulder. The pressure should be exerted on the upward stroke and released on the downward stroke. You are pushing the blood up towards the top of your arm. Repeat for other arm.

Hand and wrist sequence

Place the thumb of your left hand on the knuckle of your right hand. Drain from each knuckle to the wrist in long smooth strokes. Repeat until you have 'drained' the entire hand and wrist. Firm pressure is required from the start of the stroke to the end of the stroke. Repeat for other hand.

Stomach and chest sequence

Place flat hands on your stomach and massage both hands in large circles over your entire torso. The right hand travels anti-clockwise and the left hand clockwise. Strokes are firm.

Lower back and spine sequence

Stand with your legs shoulder-width apart. Place your hands on your hips with fingers in front and thumbs on the back. Press your thumbs firmly into the spine and lower back and move in deep, firm circles. Cover as much of the spine area as possible.

Thigh and buttock sequence

In a sitting position, with your leg supported on the side of the bed or bath, or with pillows, use flat hands to work in firm circles over the entire buttock and thigh area. Once the flesh becomes warm and slightly pink, clench your fist and continue with the firm circles. Work gently at first and build the pressure up slowly.

Calf and foot sequence

Placing both hands flat on the tops of your feet, brush them up towards your knees in long, firm strokes. Repeat for 30 seconds using a quick, rapid movement. Move your hands to the back of your leg and press the flesh firmly, lifting it and pushing it alternately. Work the flesh backwards and forwards, being careful not to burn it.

Now that you are aware of all the body care treatments that are a required part of the Detox Your Life programme you can plan the timing of your own programme. Ensure that you carry out these activities on a daily basis (except where recommended otherwise). Create a checklist to make sure that nothing has been missed.

Wring, pull, squeeze and stretch your flesh to create a new detoxed you.

STEP 19
Banish electromagnetic fields

Detox geopathic, electronic, magnetic, microwave, metallic and ozone stress from your life and live 'charge-free'.

The influence of technology on our lives is incredibly liberating. We can get in touch with people via mobile phones wherever they are, we can microwave our food in a fraction of the time it takes to cook conventionally. The television brings us news and entertainment, and when we turn in for the night we snuggle into warm sheets thanks to an electric blanket. We are woken on request by our radio alarm chirping at our bedside and we shower and then style our hair using electric dryers and heated curling tongs.

Life could hardly be made easier but all this convenience comes at a cost. We already have natural electromagnetic radiation from the sun and earth but reports say that we are now bombarded with 150 million times more electromagnetic signals than our grandparents were.

You only need to drive under an electricity pylon and hear the static on your radio to experience the effect of an electromagnetic field. Turn the radio on near a hairdryer and you will get interference. Listen to the buzz on a battery-operated radio when the washing machine does its spin cycle two floors away. These are all examples of electromagnetic radiation travelling through our day-to-day lives and our bodies.

But is this bad for our health or is it just another scare story? Research suggests that it is bad and it is also a contributory factor in many, many illnesses, diagnosed or otherwise. Roger Coghill is a leading expert on electropollution and lectures frequently on the subject. His view is that our bodies have their own electrical frequencies involved in growth, repair and cellular renewal. He believes that electric fields from machines and mobiles, microwaves and so on all have a detrimental effect on our own personal frequencies. According to his research, it is the alternating current – or AC – electric field that is dangerous to us and this exists whenever an appliance is plugged in or fully charged.

It has been suggested that conditions such as ME, lethargy, headaches and some cancers are the result of our bodies' inability to repel electric fields – some people also believe that electromagnetic fields disrupt our immune systems.

Roger Coghill believes that we are resilient to short-term exposure; we should simply reduce all constant or longer-term exposure.

Here are some ways in which you can reduce your long-term exposure:

- It seems that sleeping with a radio alarm can increase your exposure at the very time your body needs all its faculties, as our cells are repaired while we sleep. General advice is to move the radio alarm so that it is at least 4ft (1.2m) away. Alternatively, you can resort to a good old-fashioned wind-up alarm clock and get some charge-free rest! (Some say long-term exposure is most likely to happen whilst you are sleeping in one spot for approximately seven hours per day.)

- Electric blankets are reportedly tantamount to actually getting into an electromagnetic field! Even when the blanket is turned off you are still lying on a metallic grid and this will upset your own natural electric fields. Ditch the blanket and just put on a warmer duvet or snuggle up closer.

- Mobile phones are reputed to cause brain tumours. If you really need to use one, the best advice is to get an earpiece which reduces the exposure of your head to the phone, or enclose the whole phone in a shield which is available from mobile phone stores.

- Unfortunately, our parents were right all along . . . 'Don't sit too close to the television' is an all-too-familiar memory from childhood and we have probably shouted the same phrase at our own offspring. Well, we do tend to use the television for longer periods than any other household item and advice suggests that we should sit no closer than 4ft (1.2m) from the screen. Televisions emit ten times as much electromagnetic radiation as computer screens do, so we should heed our parents just this once! Computer screens can give out negative ions, so make sure you work at least 1.5ft (50cm) from the screen and take regular breaks.

- The jury is still out on microwaves but it is commonly believed that you shouldn't spend too much time close to one, once it is turned on. It's also best to leave your food for a few minutes before tucking in – a useful piece of advice anyway as food is generally too hot to eat immediately. You can check the security of your microwave by holding a radio near the door when it is turned on. If there is inter-ference then there is likely to be leakage; repairs must be made or the appliance should be replaced.

Whatever the facts, it seems to make sense to reduce the rays.

STEP 20
Detox your finances

Make your money work for you, detox the doubt and know the future of your finance. It sounds ghastly, I know, but sorting things out can be worth it.

Most of us worry at some time or other about money. Do we have enough? Have we spent too much? Did we get value for money? Did we save any or have we wasted some?

Well, the best way to prevent yourself being worried silly and using unnecessary energy on something that may not be as bad as it seems is to detox your finances.

Take a day and look through your bank statements, cheque books, paying-in slips, salary cheques, credit cards and any cash lying around.

Even if you only work out how much you actually have in your account at any one time you could save yourself several pounds per month in unauthorised overdraft facilities. Banks are very good if you keep up a dialogue with them. They simply don't like it if you disappear, as, quite rightly, they don't know what you are intending to do with your (or their) money. They cannot read minds!

'Putting money by' is an old-fashioned concept but it can also save you many pounds in credit card interest rates. Interest rates are very competitive and you may find that you can transfer your debt to a card that will give you six months at a much lower interest rate. And, of course, if you pay off your credit cards before the five-week or four-week interest-free period ends you can actually get free credit for 30 or 40 days!

If you aren't overdrawn, and have money in your account most of the time, you may not be getting the best interest rate. Speak to your bank and ask if there is an account that will earn more money for you.

Check your bank charges. Charges are often attached to your account for no apparent reason and if you don't keep a close watch then you may be paying more than you need to.

Setting up direct debits doesn't cost anything and they take out the monthly stress of having to sit down and pay your bills. All you need do is look at your monthly bank statements to see that all the charges are being taken care of and you need never get into arrears or be cut off just because the bill slipped down the back of the fridge.

File your personal and household bills. Often the only reason you don't take up the offer of 'cheaper home insurance' or lower cost phone bills is because you cannot be bothered to find the previous bills to check if you would actually save anything. If all your bills are in order and you can access them easily, you can make changes simply and save money without any hassle.

Finances often terrify people. Yet, with only a few hours of effort, you could be totally on top of everything, saving more, and making your money work harder for you.

STEP 21
Look into the future

See yourself in a positive light and detox your life of doubt and uncertainty; talk and think your way to the success you deserve.

Affirmations and visualisations are a brilliant way of

feeling good about yourself, both immediately and in the long term. Feeling down in the dumps can be transformed into feeling positive and proactive in a matter of moments. When you have got into the habit of using affirmations and visualisations, feeling down becomes a thing of the past.

Affirmations

During the detox you can affirm your ability to complete the programme and you can visualise just how 'clean' you will be when you have finished.

You often hear people say: 'If someone tells you something often enough, you really start to believe them.' Well, that's just what affirmations are – telling yourself something, anything, so often that you really believe it, and if you believe something then it becomes real.

Affirmations don't have to be grand or extraordinary, they just have to help you. To start making affirmations you need to think about what your goal is, what you want to happen or what you want to do. It can be on any level: personal, job, home, relationship, money – anything. It is probably better to start with something small. Giving up your job and living on a tropical island might be a little too adventurous for starters! In any case, if you change something small it always leads to something bigger.

Affirmations must be positive and should be kept short. The sorts of things you might want to affirm during the detox would be:

I have a healthy body.
I am happy with my body.
I am cleaning my body.

This is my month, I will enjoy looking after myself.
I deserve to indulge myself this month.
I am feeling great.
I am feeling energetic.
I have succeeded with my own personal detox.

You get the idea. Now, all you have to do is repeat these to yourself or out loud. You should say them whenever they come into your mind – you can say all of them or just one of them. As you are saying your affirmations you should give them positive energy, feel good about saying them and smile. You should believe that they are real, they exist and that they have come true or are coming true for you. If there is a time when you say your affirmations and you feel any doubt or negative feelings then immediately say them again, this time with all the positive belief that you can muster.

If you find it difficult to remember your affirmations just jot them down on the bottom of your 'to do' list, your shopping list or in your diary. Then, each time you see them, say them to yourself two or three times.

Affirmations are completely personal. No one needs to hear them or even know that you make them. The only rule is that they just have to be what you want:

I deserve more money.
I am going to get a better job.
I am great.
I am fun to be with.
I am going to ask him/her out.
I will tell him/her that I don't agree.
I will have more time for myself.
I won't let them get to me.
I am successful in everything I do.

Visualisations

Visualisations are just the same as affirmations but you make a mental picture of the thing you want to happen. You need to create a clear picture of the object, person or situation in the way that you want it to be. Picture it in the present, not the future. This way you can see things happening, rather than waiting for them to happen. Include as many details as possible so that it is as real as possible. As with affirmations, you should bring this picture to mind as often as you can. Keep the thoughts that surround the picture positive and full of energy.

Visualisation should be a pleasant and uplifting process. If it's tiring or exhausting, it defeats the object. The more you visualise your situation, the more it becomes a real part of your life.

Affirmations and visualisations can help you reach your goals and achieve success. When you have been doing them for a while you will notice subtle changes in your mental state, and your friends and colleagues will say how much more positive you seem.

Say after me: 'I feel completely detoxed of doubt and indecision. I can do anything I want to if I put my mind to it . . .'

I can do anything I want to if I put my mind to it . . .

I can do anything I want to if I put my mind to it . . .

I can do anything I want to if I put my mind to it . . .

STEP 22
Get support from your surroundings

Why don't we design our homes so that we bring health, wealth and happiness into our lives, instead of just putting up a patterned border and bunk beds in the children's room?

We spend huge amounts of money on our homes. It is in our culture to spend time making our day-to-day lives more enjoyable. We choose colours we like, we rebuild to knock rooms together or extend into open space, we design our gardens for optimum appearance and minimum effort, we search antique shops to find the ultimate doorstop . . .

There are many other cultures that follow their own sets of rules and operate in much the same way. But some of these cultures attach deeper significance to their surroundings and the effects that they have on people. In Tibet and Vietnam they follow 'phong thuy'; in the Philippines, Indonesia and Thailand they follow 'hong sui'; and in Japan, Hawaii and India they believe in 'vaastu Shastra'.

The Chinese use the rules and science of 'feng shui' (pronounced 'fung shway' or 'fung shoy'), many of which are being introduced to Western culture. Feng shui owes its popularity to our increasing desire to get the best out of our homes and, more importantly, to become happier, healthier and wealthier individuals. Most British people find it hard to admit to wanting to make money, be successful and become prosperous. But feng shui allows this and supports the desire to make the most of what we have.

The two Chinese characters 'feng' and 'shui' literally mean 'wind' and 'water'. This reflects the fact that feng shui is concerned with earthly rather than spiritual influences. Feng shui is not a religion or an art but a science. There are strict rules of application and, along with the overall philosophy, there are many tools, techniques and exercises to be used when introducing feng shui principles into your life.

Simply put, feng shui is about getting positive energy into your life, keeping it there and using it to its optimum, and then allowing all negative energy a free route out of your life. Keeping up a constant flow of good energy, without any blockages, should bring you health, wealth and prosperity.

There are several schools of feng shui and you need to choose the one that suits you best. (There are many books and magazines that you can read to find out the basics.)

The best way to ensure that you are following feng shui principles is to get a consultation done. These can be very expensive but if you get a fully qualified practitioner, who has studied for many years rather than done a few weekend courses (see Useful Addresses), the results of the consultation will undoubtedly be worth the initial outlay.

Alternatively, you could write to a local school of feng shui and ask to become one of the students' projects that they need to complete during their studies.

Whilst you are deciding how to introduce feng shui into your life, here are some simple tools for you to use that can start you on your journey.

As we said earlier, feng shui has a lot to do with the flow of energy. In order for energy to flow, all blockages or obstacles need to be removed. Anything that might shut it off, redirect it or prevent it from entering every part of your home should be rectified. In the same way, anything that speeds up the energy, or results in there being too much energy, should also be carefully looked at so that a balanced flow is maintained.

Stand outside your house on the street, facing your front door, and imagine that you are the positive energy. Look around and ask yourself if there is anything that is blocking your access to your home. Is there a tree across your front door? Is your front door old and dirty? Is the drive long and funnel-like so that too much energy speeds up towards the door and overpowers it? Or is the path just long enough for the energy to arrive at the door, ready for entry? Does the front door work? If it sticks, get that fixed. Does the hallway lead you through the house or is there a wall in the way that blocks the flow? Is there a door you never use or that is blocked by a piece of furniture? If so, clear the block and open the door – let the energy flow in.

Check that there are no mirrors facing each other. As a rule, that just bounces energy backwards and forwards and interferes with the flow. Move the mirrors so that they don't reflect on each other but reflect the energy out into the house and encourage its path. Hang all doors so that they open into the rooms and not back out into the hall or corridor, so that when you approach a room you naturally flow into it. Check that the back door is not blocked and opens outwards so that all energy, once it has passed through the house and has been used, can exit freely. Check, however, that the front door is not in line with the back door as you will find energy entering your home and then zooming straight out the back before it has circulated its beneficial properties.

Once you have completed your journey through the house, you will be more aware of your home's dynamics and may wish to make some changes to get the optimum flow. You have now completed a few basic steps towards implementing feng shui into your life; you have detoxed the negative energy and promoted the positive energy. Well done.

> **Goodbye to _sha_ (negative energy) and
> hello to _chi_ (positive energy).**

STEP 23
Nourish all your personal elements

We are not talking about fire, water, wood, metal or earth but we _are_ talking about the personal elements that make you. Detox every element of your life that drains, annoys or irritates you and boost the areas that make you grow.

We all have aspects of ourselves that we use every day, aspects that only our friends know, and aspects that we keep very much to ourselves.

Making sure we nourish all these aspects is important – concentrating on certain areas may mean that other areas get neglected and go stale. The best way to think of this is in terms of roles or job titles:

Deirdre the daughter
Deirdre the sister
Deirdre the friend
Deirdre the accounts' clerk
Deirdre the godmother
Deirdre the potter
Deirdre the knitter
Deirdre the socialiser
Deirdre the decorator
Deirdre the dog-lover
Deirdre the film buff

If Deirdre spends all her time being the friend then she will get a bit stale and long for the stimulus of the other aspects of her life. If she's working very hard then Deirdre the accounts' clerk will be too dominant and she will become too work-focused.

Just being aware that there are many aspects of your life that all need activating from time to time means that you will achieve a healthy balance.

Today you should spend some time working through your list of personal elements. Don't forget to search right back to the things that have gone so stale that they have dropped off. For instance, if you played football at school and enjoyed it but haven't played since you became a mother, then remind yourself of that element. You may not need to activate Deirdre the footballer as often as, say, Deirdre the sister, but it may enhance your life nevertheless.

Write your list and check how many times in the last day/month/year you have activated your elements. Then assess if some need activating more or less frequently.

Nourish them and watch them grow.

STEP 24
Exercise

Exercise is incredibly important – the amount of physical and mental detoxing that can result from a small bout of exercise is amazing.

Whatever form of exercise you choose you should treat it as something that you deserve and that enhances your life. It is too easy to think of exercise as hard work and a chore, something that both your mind and body have to endure, when actually both your body and mind love exercise and need it to function efficiently.

There is no excuse for not doing any exercise, especially if you are a member of a gym and don't make the most of it. Would you pay £565 for a swim or £360 for a single workout? No? Well, if you don't use a membership that you already have, that is probably exactly what you are doing. How embarrassing. Get out there now and get your money's worth.

Exercise can do all of the following, and in a relatively short space of time. I use this list a lot – it really does the job of convincing the 'unbeliever' that exercise is worth taking up. Exercise can:

- speed up the metabolism
- relieve constipation
- increase stamina
- increase the body's ability to fight infection
- help prevent heart disease
- prevent osteoporosis
- reduce the risk of breast cancer
- decrease the risk of colon cancer
- lessen arthritis pain
- lower blood pressure
- control cholesterol
- burn fat
- burn calories
- alleviate PMS
- help you stop smoking
- reduce alcohol consumption
- relieve depression

- release anxiety
- reduce stress
- improve sexual performance
- enhance self-esteem
- heighten sense of well-being
- improve mental sharpness
- increase IQ performance
- improve concentration
- enhance creativity
- improve outlook
- increase productivity
- increase job satisfaction
- improve flexibility
- preserve muscle
- improve circulation
- increase mobility
- improve memory
- improve reaction time
- deepen sleep
- increase energy
- lengthen life
- make you happier

Just 30 minutes of exercise every other day and you should feel the benefits within two weeks.

It is time to stop using the car so much and get out and walk. Stop thinking that exercise is difficult and remember that fitness is essential. With increased energy levels, everything you do around the house and the office will become less effort and more invigorating.

Stop driving to the corner shop. Stop staying in all day on Sunday and watching television. Stop putting off going to the gym. Stop deciding to get fit tomorrow. Stop trying to avoid long walks. Stop eating too much. Stop ignoring the opportunity to get fit and healthy, become full of energy and be raring to go.

Exercise costs nothing; it can be done at any time of the day or night; it can be done whilst you are doing everyday chores; and it has many, many benefits. Now that you have enough reasons, you should do at least 30 minutes every day during your detox programme. Not only will this help to keep you fit and toned but it will also ensure that your metabolic rate does not decrease or your circulation become sluggish.

Little and often is also much better then spending two hours on vigorous exercise every two weeks. This is likely to tire you out more quickly. You will not build up any benefit from your exercise, as it happens too infrequently, and this will be discouraging and you will probably give up. If you exercise for 30 minutes every other day, it doesn't interfere with your routine too much, it's over before you get bored and you will notice the benefits after just a few days. You are also much more likely to get inspired to start doing 30 minutes every other day until you build up to a level of exercise that naturally suits you and your lifestyle.

Getting started is the hardest part. Think about how your day works and how you can slip in the exercise without even noticing. Here are some examples:

- If you normally drive to pick up the children from school, then walk.

- You could jog whilst vacuuming the house or stretch for five minutes whilst dusting.

- If you are going to be sitting in a meeting for several hours, go to the meeting room via the longest route and run up the stairs several times before sitting down.

- In the evening, whilst watching the television, you can lift and lower your legs or tense and relax your stomach muscles several times.

- When everyone is out of the house, put some music on and dance for 30 minutes – this feels great and is good exercise as well!

- Don't go out to a bar – go to a nightclub and dance.

- Go rollerblading rather than walking on Sunday.

- Don't watch the kids in the pool, get in there with them.

- Sit in the bath and do stretches from side to side or scissor your legs together and apart using the water as weights – be careful not to splash too much!

Of course the more traditional methods of exercise are still very valuable (joining a gym, going to exercise classes, playing sport, jogging, etc) but if you have tried all these and not found your natural form of exercise, don't be discouraged. Set yourself a challenge to find the most unusual form of exercise you can, and do it for 30 minutes every other day.

If you are the type of person who likes to follow sequences, get a video exercise tape of someone you like and admire. Gradually build up the amount of time you spend following the exercise routine until you can do the whole tape without blinking.

Alternatively, the next few pages will take you through an elementary routine that you can do yourself.

Exercise sequence

- Warm up by walking up and down ten steps or stairs for five minutes at a normal pace.

- Sit on the floor with both legs out in front of you and feet pointing upwards. Slowly lean forward, with your back straight, to touch your toes. Feel the stretch in your lower back. Hold the stretch and then repeat five more times. Remember, do not bounce the stretch. Just pull forward until you feel your muscles working.

- Now move both legs apart so that they are still out in front of you but spread out to either side. Place both hands flat on the floor between your legs and slowly walk them forward – keeping your back straight – until you can feel the stretch in the inner thigh and along the back of the legs. Hold and then repeat five times to stretch your legs thoroughly.

- Bring your legs back together and shake the stretch out.

- Stand up and then complete the stretch by placing your feet shoulder-width apart and walking your hands down your legs until you can feel the stretch in your lower back and along the back of the legs. Hold the stretch and repeat five times.

- Still standing, lift your right foot behind you, with your knee bent. As you lift your right foot, hold it with your right hand and feel the stretch through the front of the thigh. Repeat five times. Then, if you wish to increase the stretch, you can push your thigh out behind you, being sure to keep your hip straight and not twisted.

- Repeat for the other side and lower your foot to the ground on completion.

- Stand with your feet shoulder-width apart and alternately lift your left leg and left arm up and out to the side, then your right leg and right arm up and out to the side. Repeat ten times on each side.

  NB: Keep your arms and knees slightly bent.

- Standing in the same position as before, clasp your hands in front of your nose with your arms slightly bent. Keeping your shoulders relaxed, twist slowly from side to side. The stretch will increase gradually and you should stop when you can see directly behind yourself. Feel the stretch in your stomach and waist muscles. Repeat ten times on each side.

- Walk on the spot for five minutes, making sure that you bring each knee up to hip level. Swing your arms up and down in a marching motion. Bring your hands up to shoulder height.

- Walk on the spot for five minutes, bringing your knees up and out to the side to hip level. Clasp your hands in front of you, with your forearms close together. As you step, lift your arms and lower them, without letting your arms drop below shoulder height.

- Facing forward, twist your head slowly from side to side. Look over your right and left shoulder alternately, hold the stretch for a moment and release. Then look over the other shoulder.

- Standing with your feet shoulder-width apart, hold the back of an upright chair and lower your body until your knees are bent at 90 degrees, hold the position for a count of five and rise up slowly. Repeat 15 times. Remember to clench your buttocks and thighs as you raise and lower your body.

• Take a bag of sugar or a can of tinned food, 1–2lb (0.5–1kg) in weight. Bending your knees, lean forward and place your left hand on your left knee, keeping your back straight. Take the tin or bag in your right hand and bend your right arm to a right angle. Lift the weight out and backwards, keeping your shoulder still, and just moving your arm at the elbow. Repeat the movement 15 times and then swap sides.

All these exercises, except the jogging, should be slow and deliberate. You should use your body weight as resistance to increase the effectiveness of the exercises. You can build up the repetitions as soon as you become comfortable with the programme. Do them for as long as you wish and aim to build up to doing your exercises for 30 minutes every day.

Watch your posture whenever you take part in exercise programmes. Incorrect posture will prevent your muscles from achieving peak elasticity and flexibility. Allowing your body to adapt to an incorrect position when you are fit and healthy will also cause huge problems when you are older and less flexible.

Posture is also an important factor in efficient organ function. We are all designed so that our internal organs have sufficient space to operate efficiently. If we change this spacing by putting on weight, losing a lot of weight, sitting with our bodies squashed, or slumping whilst we eat, then our organs need to adapt. This will lead to problems such as inefficient expansion of the lungs whilst breathing; lack of oxygen in the body; incorrect absorption of vital vitamins, minerals and nutrients; indigestion; poor circulation; and headaches. More obvious physical effects occur as well, such as slouching shoulders, weak stomach muscles and a caved chest. Exercise will prevent all of these problems occurring and will correct any that have already set in.

Get into the habit of taking regular exercise – and make the toxins sweat a little!

STEP 25
Detox your home and workplace

Detoxing your home is part of detoxing your life. In order to detox your life, you need to assess, prioritise and then expel all the unnecessary 'stuff'. Old clothes, unwanted furniture, goods and kitchen items all count as 'stuff'. Go through all your possessions and sort them into piles of things you definitely want, things you don't want, and things you are not sure about.

Our homes are full of furniture, books, records, contents of old Christmas crackers, buttons that don't match, single socks, old school textbooks, broken bits, clothes, shoes, hats and scarves. We buy new stuff to replace out-of-date or worn-out stuff but we hardly ever throw or give anything away.

Now is the time to bag up the things you don't want. Take them to a clothing agency or charity shop, or donate them to a jumble sale that will benefit some local cause – or even experience the joys of the car boot sale. Keep what you want and put them back in their drawers or cupboards (you should have lots more space by now).

Place all the things you are not sure about in a bag, store them somewhere out of the way and apply the six-month rule: if you don't use the contents for six months, take them all to the local charity shop, dress agency or jumble sale. Other people can benefit from your detoxing, and you will benefit because you have removed all the stale unwanted goods from your home.

When it comes to detoxing your kitchen, you need to throw out all foods that have a use-by date that has passed and you need to clean the shelves before putting any of the food back into the cupboards. Introduce a system so that every time you buy new food to store, you place it behind the existing stocks. That way, you will use the food in rotation, instead of continually having to throw good food out purely because you forgot you had it!

Detoxing your office will help you clear your mind, making the energy flow and your business grow and prosper. You need to go through all the files and see if anything has been duplicated or is no longer relevant. Decide how much filing needs to be kept as current and put the rest in archive files, so that day-to-day paperwork is easier to access.

Start by 'putting your affairs in order'. Create a filing system if you don't already have one. Put invoices in date order. Find a place for an efficient petty cash record. Label files so that you do not need to open them and trawl through them just to find out their contents.

Clean the screen of your computer and wipe greasy finger marks off the keyboard.

Feng shui your desk by clearing away all the clutter from the surface. If you have a messy desk, you will have a messy business. And if you cannot see your workspace in front of you (because it's under piles of papers), you won't have a clear route forward to drive your business.

Place your workstation or desk so that it faces into a room, not directly up against a wall. Again, the rules of feng shui state that facing a wall means you have no view of the future and your progress is blocked.

Detox your handbag or your briefcase. Even the everyday things that you use without any thought can be detoxed! Look through your briefcase and remove all the old receipts and old documents that don't need to be there. Throw out all the pens that don't work and carry a pen that actually does. Put all the small change swilling about in the base of your bag into a pot. Together with all the change from down the side of your sofa, it may even add up to the price of a pint or a glass of wine every now and then! Carry one or two lipsticks that have colour left in them, instead of a selection of old fluffy ones that have snapped off and you don't wear anyway. Take a look at your personal organiser. Are you still carrying last year's diary pages? These could be filed safely at home, saving you the trouble of flicking to the wrong year every time you try to fix a meeting.

Even small things can be detoxed. Get rid of the excess waste of keys on your keyring. I recently went through mine and realised that I had had keys cut to give to three people, moved offices before handing them out, and was still carrying three outside door keys to a building I no longer worked in.

**You can detox just about everything –
it is the key to calm!**

A FINAL THOUGHT ...

Desert island desires

If someone asked you what five things you would take to a desert island (five things that would get you through the rest of your life), what would they be?

Once you decide, look at what you have written and make a note of how much attention you have paid each item on the list in the last week, month and year.

These are what you consider to be the most important things in your life, yet you probably just take them for granted and pay them little or no attention. You certainly don't nourish and develop them as much as you could. You may even have chosen something that you hadn't considered was important to you until you thought you might have to give it up.

Decide, now, to make the five most important things in your life your priority.

As you have completed a genuine landmark task by thoroughly detoxing every last bit of waste from your life, it is now time to move forward with the things you truly believe in and desire. It is time to reassess and make what is important to you REALLY IMPORTANT ...

4

A Seven-Day Dietary Detox Programme

Detoxing your life is a big enough task to take on and if you have got this far then you deserve hearty congratulations – well done.

But detoxing must also take place within, so the following pages give you the basis for a very thorough internal cleanse.

The information in Step 2 (supplements, immune-boosting herbs and minerals) will work very much more efficiently if your internal organs are fresh, clean and raring to go.

You should eventually aim to build up to a 30-day detox diet but for now, and as you have already done some amazing work in detoxing your mind, body and soul, you can start with a straightforward seven-day plan. You may even like it so much that you don't actually come off it!

While you are following this detox programme you should enjoy yourself – think of it as a week at your own personal health farm. You deserve time for yourself and you should see the programme as a treat for your body. Don't keep thinking about the things you can't have – think about all the new things you can try.

This detox programme is very specific. If something is not listed in the next few pages then it is not included in the programme. You do not need to be a whizz in the kitchen but do try to keep varying your food choices, as this will make the programme more interesting.

In the same way as you probably follow a routine in your meals at the moment (e.g. toast and coffee for breakfast, sandwiches for lunch and a pasta dish for supper), it is completely normal to fall into a routine of having a similar thing at each meal whilst you are on the programme. Just try to make the ingredients slightly different each day.

Detoxing is not just about food. There are lots of ways that you can pamper your body from the outside as well as the inside – in just seven days you will feel much healthier, much happier and much more vital.

Take each day at a time. You are probably already wondering if you can get to day 5 when you haven't even finished reading the programme through! Each day brings positive benefits for both body and mind, and each day you will feel different as your body wakes up to the pleasure of detox.

Following a seven-day detox is quite simply. Once you have made some basic preparations, you will be ready to start.

Stage 1: Preparation

First you need to do a little self-assessment.

Count how many cups of tea and coffee, or glasses of alcohol you drink in a week. If you drink more than 14 cups or glasses in total, you should cut down to a maximum of one cup of tea or coffee or one half-pint (300ml) glass of alcohol *per day* for a week before you detox.

Count how many portions of fresh raw fruit or fresh raw vegetables you eat in a week. If it is less than two per day, start eating at least two pieces of fruit and two portions of vegetables a day for a week before you detox.

Count how many glasses of water you drink per day. If it is less than four, start drinking at least four glasses of bottled or filtered water every day for a week before you detox.

You are now ready to DETOX!

Stage 2: The seven days

The seven-day programme starts with two full days of juice only. It is best to start the programme on a Saturday, as this means that you are drinking juice over the weekend and you are more likely to be able to get some rest as your body adjusts. By Monday morning you should be well on the way to detox, and you can take ready-prepared containers of detox foods to work or visit your local snack bar. If you have to eat out during the week you should be able to order quite easily – grilled salmon on roast vegetables with a pine nut crust drizzled with olive oil is utterly detox and quite delicious.

You can also make your own dishes – remember that the food lists are simply a list of ingredients. (See the suggested recipes in Chapter 5.)

Keep an open mind and you could not only detox but make some lifelong changes to your diet.

Days 1 and 2

On days 1 and 2 you must drink only fruit juices. Juicing causes a sharp rise in blood sugar so if you are suffering from low blood sugar, diabetes or candida simply follow the plan from day 3 for all seven days.

Choose from any of the following fruits: apples, grapes,

grapefruit, mango, papaya, pears, pineapple, strawberries.

When following a full day of fruit juicing you must stick to just two fruits to help the digestive system. You should juice up to 3lb (1.3kg) of fruit or four pieces in the case of grapefruit, papaya, pineapple or mango. You should also dilute the juice 50/50 with water. Make sure you drink water between juices to help wash through the system.

You are likely to feel hungry over these two days but this is normal. If you really need to munch on something you may eat seedless grapes. You could also add some grated fresh ginger if you want to vary the tastes throughout the day.

Days 3 to 7

- Drink a cup of hot water (filtered or bottled still water) and lemon juice first thing every morning.

- During the day you must drink 3 pints (1.5 litres) or equivalent measure of water.

- Have one glass of carrot or beetroot juice.

- Eat at least three meals every day from the food lists.

- Have at least one portion of rice every day, preferably short-grain brown rice.

- Have at least four portions of vegetables – three should be raw.

- Have at least three portions of raw fruit.

- Have at least three portions of salad.

- Have at least one portion of non-dairy yoghurt, cheese or milk every day. (Non-dairy means goat's or sheep's products, rice products like rice milk or soya products like soya milk.)

• Have two portions of either pulses, nuts, herbs, olive oil or any seed oil or fish every day.

Eat as much as you want from the following lists, except potato which you should restrict to one large potato per day:

Fruit: Apples, apricots, bilberries, blackberries, blackcurrants, blueberries, cherries, cranberries, currants (dried and fresh), damsons, dates, figs, gooseberries, grapefruit, grapes, green-gage, guavas, kiwi fruit, lemons, loganberries, lychees, lime, mangoes, melons, mulberries, nectarines, olives (green or black), passion fruit, papaya, peaches, pears, pineapple, plums, pomegranate, prunes, quinces, raisins, raspberries, rhubarb, strawberries, sultanas.

Vegetables and pulses: Artichokes (globe or Jerusalem), asparagus, aubergine, beans (French, runner, broad, butter, haricot, mung, red kidney), bean sprouts, beetroot, broccoli, Brussels sprouts, cabbage (red, savoy, white, winter), carrots, cauliflower, celeriac, celery, chicory, Chinese leaf, courgette, cucumber, fennel, kohlrabi, leeks, lettuce (all types), marrow, okra, onions, parsnips, peas (all types), chick peas, peppers, plantain, potatoes, pumpkin, radishes, spring greens, swedes, sweetcorn, sweet potatoes, squashes, turnips, watercress, yams.

Nuts: Almonds, brazils, cashew, chestnuts, hazelnuts, macadamia nuts, pecans, pine nuts, walnuts.

Herbs, spices and seeds: Alfalfa, basil, cardamom pods, cayenne pepper, chilli pepper, chillies, coriander, dill, fennel, ginger (fresh and powdered), marjoram, mustard (grain, not powdered), parsley, pepper (fresh ground), pumpkin seeds, rosemary, sage, sesame seeds, sunflower seeds, tarragon, thyme.

Non-dairy: Goat's cheeses, sheep's cheeses, goat's milk, sheep's milk, tofu, goat's yoghurt, sheep's yoghurt, soya milk, rice milk.

Fish: Cod, crab, haddock, halibut, lemon sole, lobster, plaice, herring, mackerel, pilchards, prawns, salmon, sardines, scampi, shrimps, skate, trout, tuna.

Drinks: Water (hot, cold, fizzy, spring, bottled), herbal teas (any), lemon juice in water, honey in water.

Oils and miscellaneous: Olives, olive oil, sesame oil, grapeseed oil, walnut oil, apple cider vinegar, balsamic vinegar, miso, tofu, quorn, seaweed, rice cakes (unsalted), tahini (available from most health food stores – use 'light' tahini, made from sesame seeds that are hulled before being ground, or 'dark' tahini which simply means that the hulls have been left on; make sure that your tahini is unsalted).

In order to get a healthy spread of nutrients you must have some of each of these food groups every day. Missing out on one may mean that you begin to feel lethargic, as something is missing from your daily requirements. You do not need to have everything for every meal but a sensible combination might be: fruit for breakfast, salad for lunch, roast vegetables and rice for supper, nuts for a mid-morning snack, and goat's cheese and rice cakes for dessert. Try to vary this as much as possible but make sure you eat it all! It is important to include raw foods as well as lightly cooked foods, because raw foods provide bulk and roughage which will increase your body's ability to detox.

Help yourself to anything from the food lists.

The following foods are *not* permitted as they are likely to be too high in potassium or sodium, *too* fatty, *too* acidic, *too* alkaline, *too* irritating to the stomach, or they are common 'intolerance' foods or just plain bad!

What you cannot have: Tomatoes, oranges, spinach, lentils, avocados, bananas, peanuts, mushrooms, bread, cow's dairy products, sugar, caffeine, chocolate, salt, pasta, any flour-based products, alcohol, eggs, meat or poultry.

The detox rules

The detox programme is very specifically named – it is a *programme and not a diet*. A portion is the same as a heaped tablespoon. Each meal will include a combination of at least three portions of either rice, vegetables or miscellaneous foods. Each meal should be a full plate or bowl. If you get hungry at any stage, you must eat something (especially in the first half of the programme, as your body adjusts). You are likely to think that you are eating more than you should – this is normal and correct.

Vegetables, fruit and rice provide carbohydrates and fibre, whilst fish, oil and nuts are good sources of protein and fats. You must include at least two portions of foods such as olive oil, cashew nuts and oily fish every day otherwise your programme will lack the necessary balance (you are not eating any of your normal fats so adding healthy oils is crucial). If you just eat vegetables, rice and fruit you will become tired and your detox process will slow down to a standstill! Where possible, choose organic foods.

The detox programme is not calorie-counted but calories are a good way of demonstrating how much you need to eat. Calories are the method we use to measure energy in our food. The average female should eat around 1600 calories per day and never go below 1000 calories even when dieting. If our calorie intake is reduced below 1000 calories we are not providing sufficient energy for our bodies to operate and we go into starvation mode – our bodies store fat for times when they need it, the metabolism slows down, and we become weak and lethargic. It is imperative that you do not let your intake go below the recommended 1200 calories per day. The detox will only work if you keep all your organs and systems functioning healthily.

There are many occasions when you are likely to get the munchies so be prepared and have some dried fruit or nuts to hand, or carry unsalted rice cakes with some home-made hummus.

Cooking techniques
Try to cook your foods as little as possible on the detox programme. The less heat the food is subjected to, the more nutrients will remain. Obviously all fish dishes need to be cooked thoroughly but vegetables should always be eaten 'al dente'. Techniques such as light steaming, par-boiling, microwaving, stir-frying, flash-frying or grilling are much better than boiling or slow cooking, as these will reduce both flavour and nutrients.

Get creative in the kitchen
You now have an extensive list of individual fresh foods. All you need to do now is start using your imagination. These individual items can be combined to make many delicious dishes – without any additives or preservatives.

Entertaining
Having friends for supper is easy on the detox programme. For example, fish, olives, herbs and vegetables are all on the

list so you could serve grilled fish with a herb and olive crust on a bed of chargrilled vegetables drizzled with olive oil – a dazzling gastronomic success! There are many other combinations (see Chapter 5) that your guests will find it hard to believe are 'detoxing' recipes.

The inside and the outside

The detox programme keeps your body in the best possible condition from within. The nutrients from the foods, the internal cleansing actions of the rice, lemon water and fluids, and the enhanced functioning of the eliminatory organs, all provide a full internal cleanse. There is also much you can do to enhance the vitality of your body and mind through a daily and weekly body care routine from the outside.

Daily routine

From day 1 to day 7 you must:

- Have a cold shower every morning
- Do dry skin brushing every morning
- Take 30 minutes exercise every other day
- Have ten minutes relaxation every day
- Smile or laugh heartily every day
- Exfoliate every other day
- Have one Epsom salts bath on day 3 or 4

All these techniques have been described in the 25 steps in the preceding pages so you really have no excuse not to do them. They will enhance your dietary detox and play a huge part in detoxing your life – get ready to feel totally cleansed and ready to start afresh.

Cold showers boost your circulation and give your day a kick-start – they are both refreshing and toning. Simply turn the tap to cold for one minute before jumping out and rubbing down with a towel.

Dry skin brushing/exfoliation sloughs away the dead skin cells and allows your body to 'breathe'. It clears the pores and improves the appearance of your skin; stimulates the production of sebum (which in turn helps to improve the texture and tone of the skin); and improves blood and lymph circulation (the body's own waste disposal system).

Exercise offers immense benefits – so just get out and do some! Even if it means running up and down your stairs for half an hour, just do anything that will get your pulse racing for 30 minutes every other day and you will definitely notice the difference in just seven days.

Relaxation is just as important as exercise. Spend time reading a book, listening to relaxing music, or doing some basic meditation. Just ten minutes a day put a full stop after what went before and a capital letter on what is to come.

Smiling doesn't cost anything and it is very catching. Once you've had a good smile, you can deal with anything and congratulate yourself on your successful detox.

Epsom salts baths help draw the toxins out through the body's biggest organ – the skin. Epsom salts consist of magnesium which is an essential requirement for nearly all our cellular activity. As well as cleansing the body, an Epsom salts bath will improve your circulation and speed up the elimination of toxins.

Having completed the seven-day programme, you will feel energised and invigorated. You have not only cleaned your body but you have given it a holiday and it will reward you with extra energy, clear skin and a positive glow – well done!

5

Suggested Recipes

There are many recipes you can use for the Detox Your Life programme. Here is just a small selection of brain foods* and recipes suitable for the 7-day dietary detox**. Use your imagination and experiment. There will be meals that you make and choose not to do again! But there will also be meals you create that will become a staple part of your diet long after you have finished the detox.

BREAKFASTS

*Muesli***

Sheep's yoghurt
Sunflower seeds
Sesame seeds
Pumpkin seeds
Dried apricots, chopped

Pour the yoghurt into a bowl. Mix together the seeds and apricots and sprinkle over the top of the yoghurt.

*Pears and Yoghurt***

1 pear
Apple juice
Goat's yoghurt

Peel the pear and place in a pan with some apple juice and water. Bring to the boil and simmer until the pear has softened. Place the pear in a bowl and pour goat's yoghurt over it.

*Detox Kedgeree***

Smoked haddock (undyed)
Milk (rice, soya or goat's)
Brown rice, cooked
1 teaspoon olive oil
Goat's yoghurt
Cayenne pepper or chopped parsley

Place the fish in a pan and cover with milk. Simmer until the fish is soft and can be easily flaked. Remove the fish from the milk and drain. Flake the fish and mix it with the cooked brown rice and olive oil. Place a spoonful of yoghurt on top and sprinkle with the cayenne pepper or parsley.

*Fresh Fruit Salad with Floral Jus**

Fruit salad has always been a good way to start the day and breakfast is the best time to eat fruit as it gets a clear run through the system without first fermenting on top of a meal.

The floral jus adds a twist to the salad and can be added in any strength to suit your taste.

> Fresh fruit of your choice (strawberries, oranges, apples, grapes, etc.)
> 1 tablespoon each of the following: Rose water, orange flower water, elderflower cordial
> 1 teaspoon honey

Chop the fruit into large chunks and place in a bowl. Make the jus by blending equal measures of the rose water, orange flower water and elderflower cordial (a tablespoon of each is recommended the first time you make the blend but you can mix to taste thereafter). Mix in the honey and serve over the chunks of fruit.

Banana Toasts*

This breakfast is brilliant to keep you going through a hectic morning.

> 2 slices bread (wholewheat or granary)
> 1 ripe banana
> A pinch cinnamon

Lightly toast the slices of bread so that they are warm and a light golden brown. Peel the banana and simply squash the fruit onto the toast. Sprinkle lightly with a little cinnamon to taste.

*Yoghurt Muesli**

1 tablespoon each of:
Almonds, flaked
Pumpkin seeds
Sunflower seeds
Dried dates, chopped
Dried apricots, chopped
1 small pot low-fat yoghurt

Mix the dry ingredients and store in an airtight container in the fridge for use during the programme. When having the muesli for breakfast simply mix these dry ingredients with a small pot of low-fat yoghurt and eat. Carry a small bag of the mixture with you in your handbag or briefcase as extra energy reserves.

*Boiled Egg and Soldiers**

Take a trip down memory lane and treat yourself to good old boiled egg and soldiers. Eggs seem to crop up very frequently in research on brain foods and this is a simple way to get you going.

1 egg
2 slices brown bread

Boil the egg for three to four minutes if you like a soft yolk and six to eight minutes if you prefer your egg hard-boiled. Toast the bread and slice into thin strips. Try not to add butter and salt, just chew the food and taste the nourishment.

Kick-start Kedgeree*

Half a cup brown rice
Milk (rice, soya or goat's)
1 fillet smoked haddock (a fillet each)
1 or 2 hard-boiled eggs

Boil the brown rice until tender but still a bit chewy. Meanwhile poach the haddock in a pan of milk for approximately four minutes, depending on thickness of individual fillets. When it is cooked, flake the fish and mix it with the rice. Slice each egg into eight pieces and place the slices on top of the fish and rice mixture.

Banana Fruit Smoothie*

Smoothies are usually a blend of fruit, fruit juice and milk, yoghurt or ice cream. They can be as runny or as solid as you wish. If you like to spoon out your smoothie like a yoghurt then use less fluid and if you like a runny smoothie then just add more juice or milk.

All the ingredients in a smoothie are to your own taste but ideally two pieces of fruit to half a pint of milk or yoghurt and 10ml of fruit juice.

Bananas
Peaches
Grapefruit
Fruit juices
Low-fat yoghurt
Milk (if desired)

Blend the fruit together to make a creamy base, add either fruit juice, yoghurt or milk or a combination of any of these until you get the consistency you want. Add the fluids a bit at a time and mix thoroughly so that it looks appetising and not 'curdled'.

Crispy Sardines on Toast*

This breakfast is one step on from an average breakfast and only a few steps short of a full main meal but could be eaten when you have a full morning ahead.

    3 or 4 fresh sardines, washed and gutted
    2 slices wholemeal bread
    1 tomato
    Sunflower oil to taste

Take the sardines and grill until the skins are crispy and golden. Meanwhile, toast the bread. Then slice the tomato and lie on the toast. Place the sardines on top and then drizzle a small amount of sunflower oil over the fish. Serve and wait for your inspiration to come!

Glorious Grapefruit**

    1 grapefruit
    1 teaspoon honey
    Raisins or sultanas to decorate

Slice your grapefruit in half and spoon a teaspoon of honey over the top. Sprinkle with raisins or sultanas and place under a hot grill for approximately one minute, until the honey turns golden brown and the fruit becomes chewy. Serve with natural yoghurt if desired or just plain naked!

Porridge with Dates and/or Figs*

Porridge oats
Dates, sliced thinly
Dried figs, sliced thinly

This recipe is simply a twist on normal porridge. The porridge oats should be cooked in the way you prefer – just follow the instructions on the packet.

Once ready, simply mix in the thinly sliced dates or figs or use a mixture of both. The chewy variation adds flavour and brain nutrients.

SNACKS

Whilst you are on the detox programme you should never be really hungry. If you are, either you are not eating enough or you have left a long time between meals. There are also times when you might like a light snack between meals. Obviously any of the dishes below can be made in smaller quantities, or you can eat any of the ingredients individually.

Popcorn*

Popcorn can be made as the packet instructs, but instead of making your popcorn in butter, substitute olive oil. When the corn is ready you can add further flavour by tossing the warm kernels in a mixture of herbs.

Rice Cakes**

Rice cakes should be in the larder at home as an emergency snack. Make sure you buy the non-salted version and have a selection of plain and sesame seed cakes to vary the flavour. For a special treat you can have the organic chocolate variety that I have recently discovered.

Nuts and Seeds**

Crunch your way to a clean inside. Make up a bag of mixed nuts and seeds to taste; you can also add chopped dried fruit for a little extra flavour. These are great, as they are small and will last in your handbag or desk drawer for at least a week.

NORMAL LIGHT MEALS, SALADS OR SIDE DISHES

The following recipes are suitable for everyday meals, salads or side dishes. They are quite simple and straightforward and should take no more than ten minutes to prepare, assuming the rice is already cooked.

When oily fish such as tuna, mackerel or sardines are listed use fresh where possible, but canned versions are acceptable if they are in olive oil, vegetable oil or spring water. Do not use canned fish in brine as the salt content is far too high. Remember: fresh is best.

When fruit or vegetables are listed you must only use fresh produce. If it's not in season choose an available alternative to suit your taste – there really is no excuse for canned fruit or vegetables (except canned tomatoes and they are not on the detox programme!).

Unless stated, the recipes are for one. The amounts are left open for you to assess your own appetite but each meal must be a plate or bowl *full*. Do not restrict your portion size. As the food is all fresh, it will generally keep to the next meal, so make more rather than less – *you should not be hungry on the detox programme.*

*Crunchy Red Coleslaw***

Equal portions to taste of:
Radishes, chopped
Red pepper, shredded
Cucumber, sliced in thin strips
Carrot, grated
Red cabbage, thinly sliced
1 tablespoon olive oil
1 teaspoon black pepper
1 dessertspoon lime juice
Smoked mackerel – a single fillet should be sufficient
Fresh coriander

Mix all the shredded vegetables together and place in a large soup bowl. Mix the olive oil, black pepper and lime juice together and stir into the vegetables. Slice the mackerel fillet into strips and lay them on top of the coleslaw mix. Chop the fresh coriander and sprinkle it over the fish. Serve with a *small* glass of apple juice.

Greek Potato**

1 large potato
1 chunk cucumber
1 chunk ewe's feta cheese
1 dessertspoon sesame oil
Fresh basil, chopped

Bake the potato until soft in the centre and crisp on the outside – you can start it off in the microwave and then crisp it in the oven on a baking tray for the final 20 minutes. Preheat the grill. Cube the cucumber and feta and mix together. When the potato is ready, split it open and fork into the flesh the sesame oil and chopped basil. Push the flesh back into the skins and spoon the feta/cucumber mix on top. Place the whole dish under the grill until some of the feta begins to melt.

Serve on a bed of mixed lettuce accompanied by a *small* glass of mineral water.

Roast Fennel with Tuna**

1 portion brown rice
1 tablespoon olive oil
1 fennel bulb
1 portion cooked fresh tuna or tuna strips or canned tuna in spring water
Fresh sweetcorn or baby sweetcorn
Juice of 1 lime
Fresh coriander, chopped
Freshly ground black pepper

Whilst boiling the rice, pre-heat the oven to 220°C/425°F/gas 7, pour the olive oil into a roasting tin and heat it in the oven. Slice the fennel bulb in half vertically, and when the oil is hot place the bulb cut-side down in the roasting tin. Roast for five minutes and then turn and continue to roast until the bulb is slightly browned and soft in the middle.

Flake the cooked tuna. When the rice is cooked, mix it with the flaked tuna and the raw sweetcorn. Toss with the lime juice, olive oil from the roasting tin and chopped coriander and place on a dinner plate. When the fennel is ready, place both halves on the bed of rice and tuna.

Serve with a grinding of black pepper.

Spicy Courgette (Zucchini) Grill**

Brown rice, cooked
1 large courgette (zucchini)
1/2 red bell pepper
1/2 green bell pepper
1 chunk ewe's feta cheese, sliced
Chilli powder

Pre-heat the grill. Place a hearty serving of rice in the bottom of a heatproof bowl. Slice the courgette and cook it in the microwave for 3 minutes so that it is still crunchy. Shred the peppers and mix with the cooked courgette. Put the courgette mix on top of the rice and cover with slices of feta. Place the whole bowl under the grill and toast until the cheese has browned on top.

Sprinkle with ground chilli powder (mild if preferred) before serving.

*Fennel Potato Salad***

1 portion new potatoes
1 red onion, chopped
1 fennel bulb, chopped
Olive oil
1 tablespoon pine nuts
1 portion cooked prawns
Lemon juice

Boil the new potatoes until nearly cooked, then drain and slice each potato in half. Fry the chopped onion and fennel bulb in the olive oil until translucent. Add the potato halves and fry until everything is slightly browned. Whilst browning the vegetables, lightly toast the pine nuts. When the vegetables have two minutes to go, add the prawns and the pine nuts and toss the whole salad together.

Serve with a drizzle of fresh lemon juice.

*Tuna Jacket***

1 large potato
Olive oil
1 portion tuna
2 small chicory bulbs, sliced
Balsamic vinegar

Bake the potato until soft. Pre-heat the grill. Drizzle a little olive oil over a piece of fresh tuna and grill it. Place the strips of sliced chicory under the grill for the last few minutes of grilling. Make a dressing from two teaspoons of olive oil and balsamic vinegar to taste.

Serve the tuna with the jacket potato and pour the dressing over the fish. You can also mix some of the dressing with the potato if you like.

Nut Salad**

2 tablespoons cashew nuts

2 tablespoons pine nuts

1 beetroot, cooked and chopped

Lettuce, shredded

2 tablespoons chopped fresh coriander leaves

Cucumber, chopped

Fennel bulb, chopped

Green bell pepper, chopped

4 tablespoons nut oil or olive oil

Juice of $1/2$ lemon

Toss all the ingredients together and serve. Alternatively you can serve the salad on top of a bed of brown rice or as an accompaniment to any of the main course dishes.

Sardines with Apricots**

1 portion brown rice

Fresh or canned sardines

1 portion soft goat's or sheep's cheese

5–6 dried apricots, soaked

$1/2$ green bell pepper

Nut oil (walnut, pistachio or hazelnut)

Lemon juice

Boil enough short-grain brown rice to fill a large bowl. If using fresh sardines, grill them. Flake and bone the fish, fresh or canned, and mix into the rice. Cube the cheese and add to the mixture. Dice the apricots and green pepper and add these too. Dress with a blend of your chosen nut oil and lemon juice.

Thai Carrot Soup**

Carrots
Vegetable stock cube (from a health food shop – not the
    normal vegetable stock cubes as these contain preservatives
    and additives)
Lemon grass
1 chilli
Goat's or sheep's yoghurt
Fresh coriander, chopped

Boil the carrots in water with the stock cube, the lemon grass and the chilli. When the carrots are soft, remove the pan from the heat and drain. Keep the water but discard the lemon grass and chilli. Mash the carrots or put them in a blender until you have a smooth purée. Add some of the yoghurt and remaining stock water to get a soup-like consistency as thick or thin as you like. Reheat the soup and serve with a swirl of yoghurt, topped with the chopped coriander.

*Ginger Vegetables***

1 large portion mixed swede and carrots
1 small portion beetroot
4 tablespoons water
1 teaspoon grated fresh ginger
1 tablespoon grated hard goat's cheese
Chopped fresh coriander

Pre-heat the oven to 180°C/350°F/gas 4. Slice the vegetables into thin strips. Place them in a large ovenproof dish, stir in the water and ginger, and sprinkle cheese over the top. Bake slowly for about 50 minutes or until the vegetables are tender. Serve with more fresh ginger and some coriander sprinkled on top.

*Roast Beetroot***

2 medium beetroot
Olive oil or nut oil
Fresh thyme, finely chopped
Lemon juice
Feta cheese (optional)

Pre-heat the oven to 220°C/425°F/gas 7. Wash the beetroot. Mix the oil and thyme to make the dressing and roll the beetroot in it. Roast for about 1 hour, until tender. Remove from the oven, squeeze the lemon juice over the beetroot, reheat for ten minutes and serve as you would jacket potatoes – perhaps with some feta cheese crumbled over the top.

*Three Bean Salad***

3oz/90g/$^1/_2$ cup kidney beans
3oz/90g/$^1/_2$ cup chickpeas
3oz/90g/$^1/_2$ cup butter beans
1 red onion
1 clove garlic
3 tablespoons olive oil
Juice of $^1/_2$ lemon

Follow the general guidelines for bean soaking (usually overnight) and cooking on the packet or box, then drain and boil together until tender (one hour). Alternatively, use ready-cooked beans canned in water or oil. Slice the onion finely and chop the garlic. Put all the ingredients into a medium bowl, toss lightly and leave in the fridge for at least one hour before serving.

MAIN COURSES

These dishes are slightly more complicated and will probably need 30 minutes' preparation. All of them would be suitable for entertaining at home, and of course they are also great for something different for your own main meals.

*Oven-baked Stuffed Peppers***

1 red bell pepper
Creamed/soft goat's cheese
Basil leaves, chopped
1 clove garlic, finely sliced

Brown rice, cooked
Olive oil
To serve:
Assorted lettuce leaves
Cucumber
Olive oil
Lemon juice
Sesame seeds (regular or ready-toasted)

Slice the pepper in two vertically, remove the seeds and place on a baking tray in a medium oven (180°C/350°F/gas 4) for ten minutes to soften. Mix together the cheese, basil, garlic and rice. Stuff the peppers with this mixture and drizzle olive oil over them. Bake in the oven for a further 20 minutes or until ready.

Serve with a large salad of lettuce and cucumber in an oil and lemon juice dressing, sprinkled with toasted sesame seeds.

Salmon with Watercress**

1 salmon steak or fillet
1 large portion watercress
Small piece red cabbage, shredded
1/2 red onion, sliced
Black olives
Small piece ewe's feta cheese
Lime juice
Olive oil

Grill the salmon until slightly browned on top but still moist in the centre. Place some watercress on a dinner plate, lightly sprinkle the red cabbage on top and then the onion. Scatter with the olives and the cheese, roughly crumbled. Place the salmon on top and dress with lime juice and olive oil.

Nutty Monkfish**

Spring onions (scallions), sliced
10 cloves garlic
Cayenne pepper
3 tablespoons walnut oil
1 piece monkfish, cubed
$^1/_2$ red bell pepper, diced
2 tablespoons crushed walnuts
$^1/_2$ pint/300ml/1$^1/_4$ cups vegetable stock
Parsley, chopped
Lemon juice

Fry the spring onions, garlic and cayenne in the walnut oil until the onions are translucent. Add the fish cubes and red pepper and fry for a further five minutes. Add the walnuts and stock and fry for another five minutes.

Serve with chopped parsley and a squeeze of lemon juice.

Roast Vegetables with a Hot Nut Crust**

2 tablespoons walnut oil or sesame oil
Selection of green vegetables: broccoli, cabbage, celery, chicory, fennel
1 tablespoon mixed nuts: almonds, walnuts, brazil nuts, etc
1 red chilli, deseeded and finely chopped

1 small slice goat's cheese or sheep's cheese

Fresh coriander, finely chopped

Pre-heat the oven to 220°C/425°F/gas 7. Heat the oil in a roasting tin in the oven. Place the green vegetables in the tin, rolling them in the oil until evenly coated. Roast until the vegetables are slightly browned and crisped.

Whilst the vegetables are roasting crush the nuts in a pestle and mortar or by placing them in a bag and rolling with a bottle, rolling pin or other hard object. Add the chilli to the nuts and sprinkle this mixture over the vegetables for the last few minutes of roasting.

When the vegetables are ready, remove them from the oven and place on a plate. Roll the cheese over the cooled roasting tin to coat it with the remaining nut and chilli mix, then place it on the plate with the vegetables and spoon any of the remaining nut mix over the entire dish. Sprinkle with the coriander and serve.

*Cod and Colcannon***

Colcannon is a popular Scottish way of serving mashed potato. This is the detox version which leaves out the cream and butter but is just as tasty and far healthier!

1 large potato

1 cod steak or fillet

1 small leek, finely shredded

1 piece green cabbage (savoy is best), finely shredded

1 clove garlic, crushed

Olive oil

Freshly ground black pepper

Boil the potato until soft. Grill the cod on both sides until slightly golden on top. Fry the leek, cabbage and garlic in a little oil until slightly browned. Mash the cooked potatoes together with a tablespoon of olive oil to loosen it. Finally, add the fried vegetables to the potato and roughly blend together. The texture of the dish will be quite rough once it has been mixed with the vegetables.

Pile the potato in the centre of a plate and place the grilled cod on top with a sprinkling of black pepper.

Smoked Haddock with Pine Nut Crumble**

1 tablespoon pine nuts
1 tablespoon chopped fresh coriander
Black pepper
Olive oil
1 fillet smoked haddock (undyed)
Courgettes (zucchini), sliced
1 onion, chopped

Crush together half the pine nuts with all the coriander and some black pepper. Add olive oil, drop by drop, until you have a stiff paste, then add the remaining pine nuts whole. Grill the haddock for five or six minutes until cooked through. Fry the courgettes with the onion in more olive oil until just golden. Spread the coriander and pine nut mix on top of the fish and continue to grill until the crumble is browned.

Put the courgette and onion mixture onto a heated plate and place the haddock crumble on top. Sprinkle with more black pepper and serve.

*Salade Niçoise***

1 tuna steak
Olive oil
Mixed herbs, chopped
Lemon juice
New potatoes
Green beans
Lettuce leaves
Black olives
Black pepper
1 clove garlic, chopped
Fresh coriander, chopped
Pine nuts, toasted

Marinate the tuna in some of the olive oil, all the mixed herbs and a little lemon juice for a couple of hours in the fridge, then remove the fish from the marinade and grill until golden.

Meanwhile, boil the potatoes until soft and the beans until crunchy. Slice the olives in half and mix them with the cooked potatoes, green beans and lettuce leaves. Pile the mixture onto a warmed plate and place the grilled tuna on top.

To make the dressing, blend olive oil, lemon juice, pepper, garlic, coriander and pine nuts and pour over the salad. Serve warm.

*Roast Vegetables with Chèvre Blanc***

Olive oil
Selection of vegetables: bell peppers (green and red), courgettes (zucchini), chicory, fennel, celery, red onions, kohlrabi

5–6 cloves garlic
Slices of chèvre blanc
Black pepper
Cayenne pepper

Pre-heat the oven to 220°C/425°F/gas 7. Put two or three tablespoons of olive oil into a roasting tin and heat in the oven. Slice the vegetables into bite-size chunks, the rougher the better. Once the oil is really hot put the vegetables and whole garlic cloves in the tin and roll them in the oil to coat evenly. Roast for ten minutes, then check for burning and roast for a further five minutes or so to suit.

Once the vegetables are cooked to your liking, place slices of the cheese on top of them and roast for a further 5 minutes or until the cheese begins to brown. Transfer the contents of the roasting tin to a bowl or plate, sprinkle with black and cayenne pepper and eat whilst hot. The garlic cloves can be eaten whole or squeezed over the vegetables.

Warming Winter Vegetables with Pecorino Romano**

Pecorino Romano is a Parmesan-type hard cheese made with sheep's milk.

Olive oil
$1/2$ onion, sliced
3 cloves garlic
Cayenne pepper
Winter vegetables (as many and as varied as you wish)
$1/2$ red bell pepper
Fresh ginger, grated

Juice of $^1/_2$ lemon

7oz/215g/1 cup brown rice, cooked

2oz/60g Pecorino Romano, grated

Heat the oil and fry the onion, garlic and cayenne for two minutes. Chop the vegetables and add them to the pan along with the ginger and lemon juice. Fry for five minutes or until the vegetables are softened but not overcooked. Add the rice to the pan and stir-fry together for a further minute. Remove from the heat, stir in some of the Pecorino Romano, and serve with the rest grated over the top of the dish.

Pumpkin or Squash Risotto*

3 tablespoons olive oil

4oz/125g shallots or mild onions, sliced

1 medium pumpkin or squash

$1^1/_2$ pints/900ml/4 cups vegetable stock

1 clove garlic, chopped

15oz/430g/2 cups uncooked brown rice

4oz/125g Pecorino Romano, grated

Heat the olive oil in a pan and fry the shallots or onions. Scoop the flesh out of the pumpkin or squash (retain the shell and put aside), cut into small cubes and add to the oil, together with a cup of stock. Cook for five minutes. Add the garlic, the rest of the stock and the rice, and simmer until the rice has absorbed all the fluid.

Place the pumpkin shell in a large pan with some boiling water and simmer until the flesh inside the shell has softened. Remove the shell from the pan, dry off the outside and pour away any liquid from the inside. Stir the cheese into the rice mixture, pile it inside the hollow pumpkin and serve with more grated cheese on top.

*Savoury Sautéed Potatoes***

New potatoes
3 tablespoons olive oil
1 small onion, sliced
1 small fennel bulb, sliced
1–2 sprigs rosemary
2 cloves garlic
1 small courgette (zucchini), sliced
1 tablespoon lemon juice
Basil, chopped
Fresh coriander, chopped

Boil the new potatoes for five minutes. Heat the oil in a pan and fry the onion, fennel and rosemary until the vegetables are soft and lightly browned. Drain the potatoes and add them to the frying pan. Add the garlic and courgette and fry for 10 minutes, until the potatoes are browned. Remove from the heat, add the lemon, basil and coriander, discard the rosemary and serve.

DESSERTS

When you are following the detox programme there is little scope for desserts unless they contain fruit. But even these should be avoided as fruit should always be eaten on an empty stomach; if left to sit on top of a full stomach it can cause acidity. Some fruit, such as melons, contain amino acids that trigger the stomach to release its contents into the intestine just 20 minutes after the food has been eaten. This is fine if the only thing in the stomach is melon, but if it contains other foods as well the result can be a disrupted disgestion.

It is best to limit your desserts to yoghurt or cheese for most of the detox programme. If you are entertaining there are many recipes to choose from, but just make sure that you keep your own portion small.

*Apple and Summer Fruit Compote***

1 large eating apple
Mixture of cherries, raspberries, strawberries, blueberries, etc
Honey
1 tablespoon sheep's yoghurt
Sesame seeds, toasted

Peel and core the apple, place in a pan with very little water and gently steam until the fruit is tender. In a separate pan simmer the summer fruits with one tablespoon of the honey until they are soft. Place the apple on a plate and pour over the summer fruits. Top with the yoghurt mixed with a teaspoon of honey, and sprinkle with sesame seeds.

*Strawberry Smoothie***

10 large strawberries or fruit of your choice
2 small pots goat's yoghurt

Put the ingredients into a blender, blend and serve as a shake.

Alternatively, if the fruit is frozen to a 'slightly hard' consistency before being placed in the blender the yoghurt will partially freeze and you will have instant ice cream.

Grilled Lemon and Almond Pineapple**

3 rings fresh pineapple
Juice $1/2$ lemon
1 teaspoon honey
Handful toasted almonds

Pre-heat the grill on a high setting. Place the pineapple rings on a baking tray, drizzle with the lemon juice and honey and grill on high. Watch continuously, and as soon as the fruit is browned remove it and serve sprinkled with the toasted almonds.

Summer Fruit Ice Cream**

Mixture of raspberries, strawberries, blackcurrants, etc
1 tablespoon honey
1 pot sheep's yoghurt

Place the fruit and honey in a pan and simmer until the fruit is soft and the honey has melted. Remove from the heat, place in a bowl and leave to cool. When cool, chill in the freezer until nearly frozen. Place the yoghurt in a blender and add the frozen fruit, tablespoon by tablespoon, blending after each addition. Serve as soon as the mixture is totally blended – it should have the consistency of soft ice cream.

Useful Addresses

The **British School of Complementary Therapy** offers a number of valuable courses and treatments:

Courses

Diploma in Aromatherapy, Diploma in Massage, Diploma in Reflexology, LaStone Therapy Training, Introduction to Homeopathy, Introduction to Iridology and Iridology Diploma, Indian Head Massage, Beginners' Aromatherapy Weekends and Beginners' Massage Weekends.

Treatments

Aromatherapy, Massage, Acupuncture, Reflexology, Cranio Sacral Therapy, Shiatsu, Alexander, LaStone Therapy.

For information, prospectus, treatment details and ordering oils, please call 020 7224 2394. Or you can reach us on our website on www.bsct.co.uk

The organisations over the page will help you find a fully qualified, registered practitioner practising that particular therapy in your area.

British Complementary Medicine Association
9 Soar Lane, Leicester LE3 5DE
Tel: 0116 242 5406

Institute for Complementary Medicine
PO Box 194, London SE16 1QZ
Tel: 020 7237 5165

Practitioners in Aromatherapy
Aromatherapy Organisations Council, 3 Latymer Close,
Braybrooke, Market Harborough LE16 8LN

Acupuncture
British Acupuncture Council, Park House,
206–208 Latimer Road, London W10 6RE
Tel: 020 8964 0222

Bach Flower Remedies
The Edward Bach Centre, Mount Vernon, Baker's Lane,
Sotwell, Wallingford OX10 0PZ
Tel: 01491 834678

Practitioners in Colonics
Colonic International Association, 16 England's Lane,
London NW3 4TG
Tel: 020 7483 1595

Space Clearing Practitioners
Karen Kingston, Suite 401, Langham House,
29 Margaret Street, London W1N 7LB
Tel: 01708 744111
email: Karen_Kingston@Compuserve.com

Practitioners in Reflexology
Association of Reflexologists, 27 Old Gloucester Street,
London WC1 3XX
Tel: 0990 673320

Meditation
Transcendental Meditation, Freepost, London SW1P 4YY
Tel: 0990 143733

The British Wheel of Yoga
1 Hamilton Place, Boston Road, Sleaford, Lincolnshire
NG34 7ES
Tel: 01529 306851

Feng Shui Courses and Information
The School of Feng Shui, 2 Cherry Orchard, Shipston on
Stour, Warwickshire CV36 4QR
Tel: 01608 664998

Index

THE BRITISH SCHOOL OF COMPLEMENTARY THERAPY

140 Harley Street, London W1N 1AH 020 7224 2394

On production of this coupon you are entitled to 5% off any course or treatment you book in either London or Stratford Upon Avon.

Brochures of treatments, courses and dates are available on request in writing to: The BSCT, 140 Harley Street, London, W1N 1AH. Or visit the website on www.bsct.co.uk

NB: Keep this coupon until payment is required and reduction will be made at time of purchase. Do not send with brochure request.

Please send a copy of your brochure to:

Name..

....

Address..

....

....

....

Telephone No. (H)...........................(W)..........................

Send to: The BSCT, 140 Harley Street, London, W1N 1AH